Stop the Clock!
Cooking

Stop the Clock! Cooking

DEFY AGING

WITH NATURAL HEALING

COMFORT FOODS

Cheryl Forberg, R.D.

Avery • a member of Penguin Putnam Inc. • New York

Every effort has been made to ensure that the information contained in this book is complete and accurate. However, neither the publisher nor the author is engaged in rendering professional advice or services to the individual reader. The ideas, procedures, and suggestions contained in this book are not intended as a substitute for consulting with your physician. All matters regarding health require medical supervision. Neither the author nor the publisher shall be liable or responsible for any loss, injury, or damage allegedly arising from any information or suggestion in this book. The opinions expressed in this book represent the personal views of the author and not of the publisher.

The recipes contained in this book are to be followed exactly as written. Neither the publisher nor the author is responsible for your specific health or allergy needs that may require medical supervision or for any adverse reactions to the recipes contained in this book.

While the author has made every effort to provide accurate telephone numbers and Internet addresses at the time of publication, neither the publisher nor the author assumes any responsibility for errors or for changes that occur after publication.

Most Avery books are available at special quantity discounts for bulk purchase for sales promotions, premiums, fundraising, and educational needs. Special books or book excerpts also can be created to fit specific needs. For details, write Putnam Special Markets, 375 Hudson Street, New York, NY 10014.

AVERY

a member of
Penguin Putnam Inc.
375 Hudson Street
New York, NY 10014
www.penguinputnam.com

Library of Congress Cataloging-in-Publication Data

Forberg, Cheryl.
Stop the clock! cooking : defy aging with natural healing comfort foods / Cheryl Forberg.
p.   cm.
ISBN 1-58333-141-7 (alk. paper)
1. Aging—Prevention.   2. Aging—Nutritional aspects.   3. Longevity—Nutritional aspects.
I. Title.
RA777.6 .F67   2002   2002074507
613.2—dc21

Printed in the United States of America
10 9 8 7 6 5 4 3 2 1

This book is printed on acid-free paper. ∞

BOOK DESIGN BY MEIGHAN CAVANAUGH

Acknowledgments

My nonconventional career path has afforded me a rich exposure to extraordinary experts in academia, research, medicine, and the culinary arts. I am grateful to my mentors along the way, who have endowed me with priceless lessons about life, health, and food.

Many thanks to Claudia Sansone, a stellar cook, writer, and friend, who was instrumental in launching this project.

I have Dr. Ron Klatz and Dr. Robert Goldman to thank for their Foreword, and John Gronvall for connecting me to them. Their belief that food and nutrition plays an integral role in health and longevity was pivotal in creating this book.

Many thanks to Dr. Nicholas Perricone for his inspiration and guidance and to Anne Sellaro for her encouragement.

I express my gratitude to my clients, patients, friends, and family, whose support and patience allowed me to complete this book, and to Laura Di Bonaventura and Tanya Henry for their support and guidance in providing the first stepping-stone to my writer's path.

A heartfelt thanks to Marie Chrabaszewski, a research dietitian at the General Clinical Research Center of Cedars Sinai Medical Center in Los Angeles. Her support, contributions, suggestions, and treasured friendship were constant from cover to cover.

The expertise and support of dietitian colleagues from the University of California at Davis and at Berkeley, Dr. Barbara Sutherland and Rita Mitchell, R.D., were invaluable.

I am obliged to my friends and neighbors, who diligently reported at designated mealtimes and patiently tasted my recipes: Father Harold Anderson, Marie Chrabaszewski, Eric Cuenin, Christian Delacruz, Maria De Sio, Shirley Elzinga, Mark Goins, Joel Goodness, Carolyn Harbor, Neil Hedin, Susan Kayden, John Pugh, Randall Riese, Brad Springer, Bill Stark, Mark Thompson, Bill Treible, and Staci Valentine.

Some of the meals wouldn't have made it to the table without talented and patient recipe testers, including my mother, Patricia Treible, and Jennifer Ford and Charlotte Niel, whose input and suggestions were greatly appreciated.

I am profoundly grateful to Oldways Preservation and Exchange Trust, an educational "think tank" whose work is based on current scientific evidence for healthy eating and sustainable agriculture. I am indebted for the guidance and inspiration of the many friends of Oldways: Dr. Ed Blonz, Dr. Kelvin Davies, Dr. David Heber, Jim Nichols, Dr. Ron Prior, Tim Snyder, Joe Vinson, and many others, but especially to Sara Baer-Sinnott and K. Dun Gifford, who made meeting most of them possible.

I am thankful to the members of the Food and Culinary Professionals group of the American Dietetic Association, the International Association of Culinary Professionals, Les Dames d'Escoffier, and the Association of Food Journalists for their knowledge, support, and camaraderie that continually inspire and motivate me.

For pulling it all together with perpetual friendship, support, and guidance for my written word, I thank Antonia Allegra and Kathleen Kennedy. And for guiding the proposal's metamorphosis into a book, I am grateful to Jane Dystel and Miriam Goderich for their belief in this project.

A special thanks to John Duff, Laura Shepherd, and Dara Stewart at Avery for continuously supporting my ideas and providing invaluable feedback and to Jeanette Egan for putting it all together with creative and insightful guidance.

Many thanks to Dr. Denham Harman, the "antioxidant pioneer," whose groundbreaking discoveries have catalyzed exponential growth in the study and understanding of the aging process.

And my most profound thanks to scientists around the world who devote their work and their lives to the study of diet and disease to afford better health for us all.

Contents

Foreword   *1*

Preface   *5*

1. How to Defy Aging by Eating
    the Foods You Love   *7*

2. Unparalleled Plums and Berries   *21*

3. Supreme Citrus and Grapes   *41*

4. Time-Honored Tomatoes   *55*

5. Aromatic Trio: Ginger, Onions, and Garlic   *71*

6. Glorious Greens   *87*

7. Sensational Soy   *107*

8. Colorful Carrots, Beets, Bell Peppers,
   Pumpkins, Sweet Potatoes, and Mangoes   123

9. Splendid Grains and Seeds   143

10. Bountiful Beans and Legumes   165

11. Fabulous Fish and Flax   187

12. Noble Nuts, Cocoa, and Tea   203

Selected References   220
On the Web   229
Further Reading   230
Shopping Sources   231
Glossary   233
Index   243

Foreword

Boomers are wrinkling. Eighty million strong, this titanic slice of the American population was born between 1946 and 1964.* From thirty-nine to fifty-seven years old, we make up 29 percent of the population. Our influential group has redefined each life-cycle stage it encounters. Our legendary youth culture personified the 1960s and '70s. In the 1980s, we emerged as the infamous "young urban professionals." And now, our powerful group is *beginning to age.* As the oldest of the Baby Boomers now approach later adulthood, we are again poised to redefine the next stage—retirement. Baby Boomers represent the largest single sustained growth group of the population in the history of the United States.

Boomers everywhere yearn for fitness and vitality with each passing birthday. But wrinkles and sagging are just a fraction of the aging repercussions we are struggling to defer. A bevy of degenerative diseases looms while we frantically cling to the health of our youth. The number of Boomers alone pushes antiaging health care to the forefront of clin-

* U.S. Department of the Census

ical medicine. In 1999, AARP conducted a poll of its membership on concerns of living to a very old age. Their chief worry was cited as declining health.

There is a new frontier on the horizon with the potential to alleviate this fear by altering the existing health-care and sociomedical structures. "Successful aging," "healthy aging," "optimal aging," "aging gracefully," however it's said, the meaning is understood.

Antiaging medicine is a specialty based on sound scientific knowledge for early detection, prevention, treatment, and reversal of age-related diseases. Its goal is to promote a healthy life span. Antiaging medicine is emerging as a highly recognized mode of health care in the twenty-first century. Based on a multidisciplinary approach, antiaging medicine embraces four key aspects of preventive health care:

○ traditional and emerging medicine.
○ exercise.
○ mental/spiritual.
○ diet.

Many of the Boomers we see are motivated, health-conscious individuals who are more likely to eat right, exercise, and take care of themselves. They have increased confidence and an overall improved outlook on life. This may not necessarily translate into a longer life, but it appears to create a more productive one. It's not surprising that these patients would have greater longevity.

Our list of cardinal rules for promoting health and longevity is:

○ Avoid stress.
○ Exercise daily.
○ Get plenty of rest.
○ Drink minimal amounts of alcohol.
○ Drink plenty of water.
○ Maintain optimal antioxidant blood levels.

Multitudes of supplement choices on the market offer a route to peak nutrition. But supplements are just that—supplemental. The first dietary key to optimal health and longevity is to increase our antioxidant blood levels the natural and old-fashioned way—through eating.

Food is a fundamental piece of the antiaging puzzle, and *Stop the Clock! Cooking* provides the essential dietary information needed for you to embark on your own journey to the fountain of youth. A professional chef and registered dietitian, Cheryl Forberg has taken the top antiaging foods and translated them into inventive and satisfying recipes that are easy to prepare. The *Stop the Clock! Cooking* Pantry provides a list of ingredients carefully chosen for their optimal antioxidant levels. The first chapter explains the theory of aging and why antioxidants are vital to slowing the aging process.

Stop the Clock! Cooking isn't just for Baby Boomers. It's a book for those who *think* about becoming older and for those who *are* becoming older. It is for everyone. *Stop the Clock! Cooking* embraces the principles of the most widely held theories of the aging process and creates a simple, approachable, and delicious venue to promote health and longevity. For anyone who truly wants to stop the clock and improve his or her quality of life, this book is a must.

Dr. Ronald Klatz is the president and Dr. Robert Goldman is the chairman of the American Academy of Anti-Aging Medicine. Dr. Klatz and Dr. Goldman have authored several books, including *New Anti-Aging Secrets for Maximum Lifespan; Stopping the Clock;* and *Stopping the Clock II: Longevity for a New Millennium.*

Preface

Until my last birthday, I never thought about getting older. But suddenly, I needed reading glasses, and missing my one-hour walk for a day or two meant stiffness in my joints. When I looked in the mirror, my reflection prompted me to add new creams and concealers to my previously meager collection. Who knew this could happen so suddenly? For the most part, I watch what I eat, and I've always been healthy. But I had to admit, I was getting *older*.

In the last two centuries, our life span has doubled from thirty-five to greater than seventy years. This is due in part to a huge drop in the infant mortality rate along with major advances in public health. We now know that genetics is a critical component of the aging equation, and experts predict major breakthroughs in our understanding of the biology of aging that will promote longevity even further.

Meanwhile, we're barraged every day with remedies that are purported panaceas for the symptoms of aging: quick fixes, shakes, pills, and creams. Since I've always advocated the preventive powers of food, I truly believed that the connection between diet and health encompassed the aging process, so I decided to dig a little deeper.

I researched free radicals, antioxidants, degenerative diseases, and more. As I read, I discovered that every day, around the world, thousands of scientists are unlocking extraordinary antiaging secrets in the most ordinary foods in our cupboards. From Tokyo to Helsinki and from spinach to nuts, fresh foods are being sliced and diced, mashed and minced, and placed not only on dinner plates but also under microscopes. And in test tubes all over, the results are surprising and affirming. Food not only has the power to heal; it specifically has the potential to reverse many symptoms of body degeneration, also known as aging.

An abundance of current findings is derived from animal studies, and human trials are under way. The breadth and global progress of existing studies convinced me of their promise. With that in mind, I wrote this book to translate the harvest of research into a feast of delicious recipes.

Stop the Clock! Cooking is an antiaging cookbook. *Antiaging* is a term used to describe anything "used or tending to prevent or lessen the effects of aging."* I can't promise that this book will prolong your life. But following the recommendations discussed in each chapter can result in benefits such as improvements in vision, memory, digestion, complexion, regularity, weight loss, and just plain old feeling great. It could change your life.

I've worked as a chef and a dietitian for clients and patients who have included royalty and celebrities, men and women, young and old, healthy and ailing. Though they indulged in *Stop the Clock! Cooking* to varying degrees, they all agreed that the flavors are a delicious diversion.

Whether you are a cooking novice or an expert, you can use the information in this book to make informed choices for grocery shopping or for ordering from restaurant menus. These foods will benefit you and your family. It's never too early or too late to begin. When in your kitchen, learn to think outside of the box. The basis for most of the recipes is the Mediterranean pantry with global influences, healthy food with an edge. A wealth of diversity in world cuisine is reflected in the sumptuous recipes that follow.

Let's get started on stopping that clock.

---

* By permission from *Merriam-Webster's Medical Desk Dictionary* © 2002 by Merriam-Webster, Incorporated.

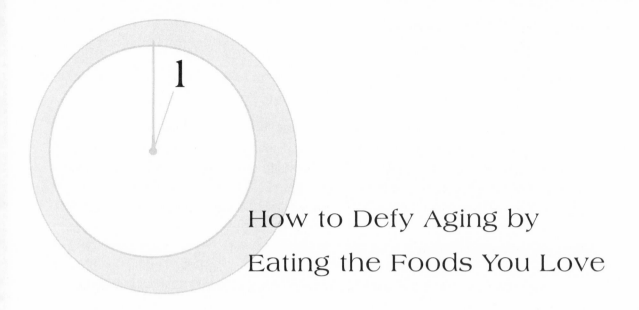

How to Defy Aging by Eating the Foods You Love

Wrinkles, fatigue, stiffness, strained vision—our greatest fears, those dreaded and inevitable effects of aging have incredibly edible antidotes. *Eat* your way to youth? Yes! Follow a delicious route to this highly desirable destination. A stressful lifestyle coupled with minimal exercise and suboptimal food choices accelerate the aging process. In tandem with our inherent genetic clock, these factors cause our bodies to weaken in many ways, making us more susceptible to illness and the physical effects of time. If choosing the right foods protected us from the ravages of aging, who wouldn't want the first bite?

It's true. The foods we eat can be our most empowering weapon in the battle against aging. Armed with keen insights into our food selections, we can minimize the levels of aging compounds in our bodies. Consequently, we may impede our aging rate while optimizing our quality of life. Growing old isn't optional, it's inevitable. But we may be able to slow the pace! Launch your journey to longevity with powerful and delicious antiaging recipes using an arsenal of healing ingredients.

THE OXYGEN PARADOX

Before heading to your kitchen to stir up a sumptuous feast, you should know just how we can defy aging by eating the foods we love. Whether or not you are an inquisitive cook, understanding the premise of what Dr. Kelvin Davies calls the "Oxygen Paradox" will make your choices not only easier but also downright seductive.

Professor of Molecular Biology and Associate Dean for Research of the School of Gerontology at the University of Southern California, Dr. Davies is a renowned expert on the aging process. In his words:

> . . . the "Oxygen Paradox" is the most delicious conundrum I know. Simply stated, the Oxygen Paradox tells us that oxygen is essential to our lives, yet extremely dangerous to live with. The reactive chemical nature of oxygen allows it to support the flames in the furnaces of a coal or gas power station, and the spark in the internal combustion engines of our cars. Our own cells use oxygen to extract energy from the foods we eat. The reactive chemical nature of oxygen allows us to "burn" proteins, fats, and carbohydrates to produce energy in our cells. Unfortunately, this same powerful oxidative potential of oxygen makes it a very dangerous ally. Oxygen causes bridges to rust, meat to go rancid, wine to sour, and potato chips to spoil. Oxygen also causes the iron proteins in our bodies to "rust," our cell membranes to go "rancid," and our DNA to "spoil." If oxygen were a proposed new food additive or dietary supplement, the FDA would have to ban it for being too toxic! By promoting "oxidative damage" oxygen contributes to the overall process of deterioration, decay, and senescence that we call "aging."

FREE RADICALS

Dr. Davies describes the most widely accepted theory on aging, the free radical theory, developed in the 1950s by Dr. Denham Harman, then a scientist at the University of California at Berkeley. Dr. Harman's theory says some oxygen molecules, called *free radicals,* initiate unfavorable changes in our bodies. He believes the changes progress, detrimentally affecting our health, with the end result being aging.

What is a free radical? It is an oxygen molecule, which is an atom or molecule with one or more unpaired electrons: either one or more extra or one or more missing. With this in mind, a free radical can be negatively charged, positively charged, or uncharged. This means it is highly reactive, causing it to react with healthy cells in its environment.

Those free radicals that are missing electrons try to "steal" them from other molecules: This is the process we call *oxidation* (of the target molecule). In contrast, radicals with extra electrons try to "donate" them to other molecules, which initially causes a reduction (of the target molecule). Both oxidative and reductive free-radical reactions, however, involve the transfer of single electrons, which means that more radicals are produced in a chain reaction. It is this chain-reaction nature of free radicals that makes them so powerfully destructive to the healthy cells that surround them.

This potentially harmful exchange of energy can have profound effects, because the surrounding cells that are affected by this change contain key elements such as DNA. The progressive changes can lead to cognitive impairment, immune suppression, diabetes, heart disease, cancer, arthritis, and other degenerative diseases. Starting to get the picture?

So where do the free radicals come from? There are many sources. We are constantly exposed to free radicals from:

- smog, pesticides, and cigarette smoke.
- medications.
- foods containing saturated fats, trans fatty acids, and processed foods.

But that's not all. There are internal sources, too. Your body is producing free radicals as you read this. Free radicals are a natural part of our metabolism. We generate them as we breathe, as we convert food to energy and as our bodies fight infection. Some of them are even beneficial.

OXIDATIVE STRESS

Internally, we store certain enzymes and the vitamins able to counteract the harmful free radicals and keep them under control. But when the number of free radicals exceeds our bodies' ability to subdue them, the power shift is called *oxidative stress*. This stress, or free radical burden, attacks healthy cells. Their accumulation ultimately results in a series of events that leads to oxidation and the process we call aging.

So how can we avoid oxidative stress? By minimizing our exposure to the external sources, we reduce our intake of free radicals from the environment. Internally, our first line of defense is our own reserve of antioxidants. The primary antioxidants in the body function as enzymes, shielding the body from oxidative damage. The enzymes exert antioxidant powers by preventing the free radical from reacting or causing harm to surrounding cells. The enzymes may be outnumbered when large amounts of free radicals are present.

One theory for deterring this shift advocates a lower-calorie diet to support oxidative balance. A low-calorie diet also lowers bad cholesterol and blood pressure and slows the body's natural decline in the level of a beneficial hormone called *dehydroepiandrosterone* (DHEA). University of Wisconsin, Madison, researchers Dr. Tomas Prolla and Dr. Richard Weindruch have found that a low-calorie diet also protects genes that normally become damaged with age, thus facilitating optimal function for a longer period.

Aside from becoming calorie counters, we can lower our caloric intake by understanding the concept of *nutrient density*. This means that, for a given serving size, some foods are higher in certain minerals, vitamins, and antioxidants relative to the number of total calories they provide.

Understanding the importance of nutrient density necessarily means that we must *minimize* our intake of nutrient-*poor* foods, such as simple sugars, to support oxidative balance. In addition to basic sweeteners, simple sugars include many refined, processed foods that may be high in caloric value but lacking in nutrients. To effectively implement this concept, then, we need to maximize our intake of nutrient-dense foods. These choices will be further discussed in the *Stop the Clock! Cooking* Pantry (page 15).

In addition to their role as a suboptimal nutrient source, simple sugars have another pro-aging detriment: They rapidly convert to glucose, our primary energy source. Glucose control is a pivotal activity of our bodies. As glucose molecules circulate, some of them attach to protein molecules in the bloodstream—a process called *glycosylation,* or *glycation.* High levels of blood glucose lead to higher levels of glycated proteins and insulin. As these levels increase, they initiate reactions with hormones and the immune system, shifting into an unfavorable gear called *inflammation.* This inflammatory state creates excess free radicals, increasing oxidative stress and producing symptoms ranging from arthritis to wrinkling.

According to Nicholas Perricone, M.D., F.A.C.N., an assistant clinical professor of dermatology at Yale University School of Medicine and author of *The Wrinkle Cure* (Warner Books, April 2001) and *The Perricone Prescription* (HarperCollins, August 2002) ". . . high levels of blood glucose result in attachment of the sugar to the collagen protein in the skin. This glycation reaction causes cross-linking of the collagen, causing the dermis to become stiff and inflexible. The result is wrinkling and sagging, two of the more unattractive conditions attributed to aging." Dr. Perricone believes that 50 percent of the aging of the skin is attributable to the effects of sugar. Dr. Perricone says that, in addition to glycation, elevated blood glucose results in an inflammatory burst in the skin cells, creating free radicals and further accelerating the visible aging process.

ANTIOXIDANTS

Meet your new line of defense. The ingredients for the recipes in this book are carefully selected to utilize nutrient-dense foods with high levels of antioxidants and lower levels of simple sugars. One group of antioxidants, known as *phytochemicals,* are chemical substances produced by plants that provide the colors, flavors, and scents of nature's bounty. Many phytochemicals safeguard the plant itself from forces of nature such as the sun's radiation. Researchers are now stirring up clues indicating that they protect us, too. Collectively, these foods are an arsenal teaming with nutritional ammo poised to wage a war against the aging compounds attacking our bodies. This is not news. The antioxidants have been there all along. We just didn't realize what a powerful punch they packed and that we are more empowered than we thought. This just may be the elusive magic bullet we've been looking for.

Although the United States Department of Agriculture (USDA) has not yet established a daily recommended intake (DRI) for total antioxidants from fruits and vegetables, Dr. Ronald L. Prior, the department's research chemist and laboratory chief, is convinced that most of us are eating less than half the amount required for optimal antiaging nutrition.

The message here is a new way of life—a style of cooking, of eating, of living. This proactive design integrates and optimizes the benefits of healthful eating to live longer and live better! One recipe per week won't stop your clock. But incorporating the recipes and recommended foods on a daily basis and, better yet, throughout the day, will make an impact. The afterlife of dietary antioxidants in our bloodstream is about six hours. (Carotenoids have a longer afterlife.) Therefore, regular intake throughout the day optimizes antioxidant levels in our bloodstream, which is the best approach from a dietary perspective. Many of these antioxidant-rich ingredients are probably on your shelves already.

Is this just another trend? No. Even though the rage seems recent, antiaging ingredients have been around for centuries. Some of them are just being discovered and others rediscovered. Ancient civilizations relied on whole grains, vegetables, fruits, and spices, many of which were believed to have specific medicinal properties. Centuries later, scientific studies have verified their healing powers. This is not a craze. As the healing properties of more foods are revealed, there will be new choices. But healing foods, *antiaging foods,* are here to stay.

With all of this information in mind, it is important to note that if you have a medical condition requiring a special diet, please discuss any concerns with your health-care provider before implementing dietary changes on your own. It is likely that he or she will be eager for you to implement part or all of the principles discussed in this book. This book is not intended as a substitute for medications or professional medical care.

WHICH FOODS ARE HIGH IN ANTIOXIDANTS?

Many research studies measure antioxidants in whole foods to determine their functionality. The ORAC measurement (oxygen radical absorbency capacity) signifies a food's ability to neutralize cell-damaging free radicals. Though we're not sure how this translates to their performance in our bodies, the chart below identifies some of the highest-ranking foods in terms of average antioxidant capacity in lab measurements.

ORAC Units[*]				
	per 100 grams (100 ml if 1g/ml), or about 3.5 ounces		*per item or serving*	
1.	Cocoa powder	50,400	1 tablespoon	3,150
2.	Cabernet Sauvignon[†]	27,400	4-ounce glass	30,850
3.	Sorghum flour	26,900	¼ cup	9,378
4.	Pomegranate	10,500	½ medium pomegranate	10,500
5.	Sorghum syrup	8,540	⅓ cup	8,540

ORAC Units* (con't.)

		per 100 grams (100 ml if 1g/ml), or about 3.5 ounces		*per item or serving*	
6.	Dried plum	5,770	1 pitted	480
7.	Blackberries	5,100	¾ cup	5,100
8.	Cabbage, purple	4,200	½ cup raw	1,479
9.	Ground flax	3,700	1 tablespoon	308
10.	Stone-ground cornmeal	3,700	¼ cup	1,233
11.	Kale	3,700	½ cup cooked	2,405
12.	Chardonnay†	3,300	4-ounce glass	3,770
13.	Blueberries	3,200	⅔ cup	2,400
14.	Plum	2,800	1 medium	2,800
15.	Red raspberries	2,700	¾ cup	2,700
16.	Strawberry	2,600	1 strawberry	217
17.	Spinach, raw	2,400	1 cup	1,290
18.	Orange	2,400	1 medium	2,400
19.	Watercress	2,200	1 cup	2,200
20.	Raisins	2,100	¼ cup	700
21.	Cherries	2,100	10 cherries	1,429
22.	Whole-wheat flour	1,900	¾ cup	1,900
23.	Cranberries	1,700	about ½ cup	1,700
24.	Dark honey‡	1,630	⅓ cup	1,630

ORAC Units* (con't.)

		per 100 grams (100 ml if 1g/ml), or about 3.5 ounces	per item or serving	
25.	Grape juice	1,563	⅓ cup	1,254
26.	Peach	1,300	1 medium	1,300
27.	Black tea	1,228	⅓ cup	1,228
28.	Asparagus	1,200	1 medium spear	240
29.	Broccoli florets	1,200	½ cup cooked	1,200
30.	Onion	1,200	½ cup chopped	960
31.	Green tea	1,125	⅓ cup	1,125
32.	Grapes, red	1,100	10 grapes	263
33.	Grapefruit, pink	1,100	½ fruit	1,100
34.	Bell pepper, red	1,000	1 medium	740
35.	Avocado, California	782	½ avocado	587
36.	Banana	500	1 medium	500
37.	Carrots	500	½ cup raw	278
38.	Pumpkin	400	½ cup cooked	326
39.	Mango	300	1 whole	300
40.	Tomato	300	1 medium	300

* ORAC values provided by Boxin Ou, Brunswick Labs; Ronald Prior and Guohua Cao, USDA Agricultural Research Service, except where noted otherwise.
† ORAC values provided by Canandaigua Wine Company of Madera, California, and Brunswick Labs.
‡ ORAC value provided by University of Ilinois, Urbana.

THE STOP THE CLOCK! COOKING PANTRY

The recipes in this book focus on nutrient-dense antioxidant-rich whole-food ingredients. It is recommended that the following foods make up the major portion of your diet.

WHOLE FRUITS

Apples
Apricots
Bananas
Blackberries
Blueberries
Cherries
Cranberries
Dried plums
Grapefruit
Grapes and raisins
Kiwifruit
Lemons
Limes
Mangoes
Oranges
Plums
Pomegranates
Raspberries
Strawberries

WHOLE VEGETABLES

Artichokes
Asparagus
Avocados
Beets
Bell peppers

Broccoli
Brussels sprouts
Cabbage
Carrots
Collard greens
Corn
Eggplant
Kale
Mustard greens
Pumpkin
Romaine lettuce
Spinach
Squash
Sweet potatoes
Swiss chard
Tomatoes
Watercress

**ANTIOXIDANT-RICH
SEASONINGS AND
FRESH HERBS**

Cumin
Dill
Garlic
Ginger
Lavender
Mint
Onions

Oregano
Parsley
Rosemary
Saffron
Sage
Thyme
Turmeric

WHOLE GRAINS AND SEEDS

Brown rice
Bulgur wheat
Kasha
Millet
Pumpkin seeds
Rolled oats
Sesame seeds
Sorghum flour
Stone-ground cornmeal
Sunflower seeds
Whole-wheat flour

BEANS AND LEGUMES

Black beans
Fava beans
Garbanzo beans (chickpeas)

Kidney beans
Lentils
Peanuts
Pinto beans

●

TRADITIONAL SOY FOODS

Edamame
Miso
Soybeans
Soymilk
Tofu

UNSALTED NUTS

Almonds
Brazil nuts
Cashews
Pecans
Pine nuts
Pistachios
Walnuts

●

OMEGA-3–RICH FISH

Anchovies
Herring

Mackerel
Salmon
Sardines
Tuna

●

OTHERS

Flaxseed
Unsweetened natural
cocoa powder

WHAT TO BUY, WHAT TO EAT

- Include small servings of lean chicken about two times per week. Egg whites are unlimited, and whole eggs can be eaten about once a week.
- Eat lean meats no more than one time per week.
- Fish can be eaten four or five times per week.
- Use organic, unsweetened, and low-fat dairy products in moderation.
- Fats should comprise 30 percent or less of total calories. If using, choose olive or canola oil.
- Avoid simple sugars, processed foods, and refined products.
- Limit use of all sweeteners. If using, choose sorghum syrup or dark honey.
- Drink no more than 1 or 2 cups of coffee per day or switch to green or black tea.
- Limit alcohol intake to one drink for women and two drinks for men daily, and choose red wine when imbibing.
- Drink plenty of water, 8 to 10 glasses each day. This is especially important because eating the recommended foods will increase fiber intake.
- Minimize salt intake.
- Eat small, frequent meals throughout the day to maintain antioxidant balance and to even blood sugar.

SPECIAL NOTES ON SORGHUM SYRUP

Whole fruits are the best choice for satisfying a sweet tooth since they have fiber, which slows the absorption of fruit's sugars into the bloodstream. Though added sweetener is not recommended for optimal antiaging nutrition, for many of us it's hard to imagine living without it. Most sweeteners, especially refined sugars, have no significant nutritional value, and they certainly don't stop the clock. They do contribute to free-radical production. Sorghum syrup has an advantage that other sweeteners don't. But first, a little more about it:

- Sorghum syrup is made from the juices of the sorghum cane plant. The juices are carefully boiled down to obtain a dark, thick, sweet, and sticky liquid.
- The dark rich syrup has a subtle caramellike flavor. It's sweeter than blackstrap molasses but not as sweet as honey or sugar.
- Sorghum syrup was an important sweetener beginning in the 1850s in the United States. As other sugars with lower production costs stormed the scene, sorghum syrup production waned, though it never ceased. In the South, it is sometimes referred to as sorghum molasses, or just molasses.

Sorghum syrup has a nutritional advantage not only over sugar but over some fruits as well. Sorghum syrup is remarkably high in antioxidants. Ounce for ounce, sorghum syrup has higher antioxidant capacity than any fruit or vegetable measured, except pomegranate. This is not an invitation to sweeten everything with sorghum syrup. Rather, it is a sweetening option that upholds the high-antioxidant profile of the foods that should be included in your pantry. Sorghum syrup is still a form of sugar, and its intake should be minimized for optimal antiaging nutrition. For occasional use, sorghum syrup is the preferred sweetener option. Honey has also shown antioxidant properties, with the darker shades, such as buckwheat honey, possessing the greatest antioxidant reserves. Sorghum syrup, however, has shown four times the antioxidant power of the darkest honey tested.

If sorghum syrup isn't available in your area, check the Shopping Sources, pages 235 to 237.

Olive Oil—The Fat of Choice

Here's why you should use olive oil:

- Its unique profile promotes increased high density lipoprotein (HDL), the good cholesterol, and a better total cholesterol profile.
- It contains vitamin E (tocopherols), an antioxidant that works against free radicals and promotes oxidative balance.
- It contains essential omega-3 fatty acids.
- It contains polyphenols, which not only enhance the aromatic taste of the oil but also have antioxidant benefits to stop the clock.

Olive oil is classified according to its processing techniques and the resultant acidity. Extra-virgin olive oil is considered to be the highest quality, whereas fine virgin, semifine, refined, and pure olive oil are other grades in descending order of quality. The structure of extra-virgin olive oil does not withstand high cooking temperatures, but it is the preferred choice of oil for an uncooked dish such as a salad or for a dressing where it is used to flavor rather than cook the dish.

Nonvirgin olive oils, such as semifine, refined, or pure olive oil, stand up to higher temperatures and are the preferred choice for cooking. Light oils with a milder flavor are better for baked goods or dishes in which a strong olive oil flavor is not desired.

Olive oil cooking spray is used in the recipes throughout this book to minimize added fat. Rather than use aerosol cans, you can easily make your own cooking spray. Spray bottles are available in health food stores and can be filled with your own fresh oils as needed. For regular baking and sautéing, fill the spray bottle with a mild-flavored oil.

Olive oil can be stored in a cool, dark place for up to 4 months. Because it is composed of highly unsaturated fats, it will turn rancid within several months after opening. Buying a large bottle with a proportionately better pricetag is not the best option if you use oil infrequently. When in doubt of your oil's freshness, throw it out and open a fresh bottle. One tablespoon of rancid oil can ruin the flavor of an entire recipe.

Special Notes on Cocoa Powder

As you'll see in Chapter 12, cocoa beans are a rich source of antioxidants. However, the naturally occurring, antioxidant-rich polyphenols in cocoa powder are acidic, which means their numbers are reduced when cocoa powder is alkalized. If this step is a part of the manufacturing method, it means that alkali is added to make what is known as Dutch-process cocoa powder. As most manufacturing techniques are proprietary, it's hard for us to discern which cocoa beans have the richest concentration of antioxidants when we are shopping for cocoa powder. One thing we can determine from the label is whether or not a cocoa product has been alkalized. If it has not been alkalized, it is referred to as natural. Look for "natural" when shopping for cocoa powder.

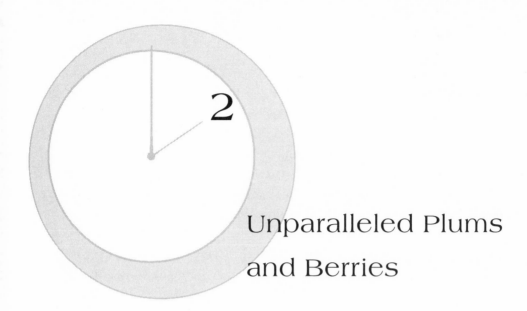

Unparalleled Plums
and Berries

It's no surprise that as we age, our brain is often first to show symptoms of aging, perhaps because it's so vulnerable to oxidation by ravaging free radicals. Fading memory, blurring vision, confusion, and waning motor coordination are all signs that the brain's abilities to function are slowing. Emerging research reveals astonishing healing powers in phyto-chemicals and their whole-food hosts.

PLUMS

When plucked from their lush tree branches, sun-drenched plums are juicy and plump stone fruit. But, like some grapes, many plums are cultivated expressly to be dried upon harvest. Formerly known as prunes, dried plums are crammed with vitamins and miner-als, including potassium, vitamin A, magnesium, and iron. They are also a source of boron, a mineral that is thought to play a key role in the prevention of osteoporosis. Dried plums also contain a number of phytochemicals called *phenolic compounds.* These rich reserves of antioxidants are thought to slow the aging process in a number of ways.

Dried plums have been the focus of a large number of recent studies related to cardio-vascular health. Results reflect a reduced incidence of heart disease in those whose diet includes five dried plums per day by slowing the oxidation process and decreasing low density lipoprotein (LDL), the bad cholesterol. Sorbitol, a sugar alcohol, contributes most of the sweetness to the dried plum's flavor profile. It may also explain the well-reputed laxative effect attributed to both prune juice and dried plums. High levels of fiber further promote regularity while helping maintain steady glucose levels.

It's not too late; have some plums to dinner, with exotic Savory Chicken Tagine with Slivered Dried Plums and Baby Artichokes or Crispy Vegetarian Spring Rolls with Shanghai Plum Sauce.

BERRIES

The latest news is that blueberries not only may prevent age-related memory and motor co-ordination impairments but also may actually promote *reversal.*

Sweetly smothering a fluffy pancake, plump and juicy in a chunky relish, or nestled in a flaky pie, there's no time of day that berries aren't a welcome addition to the menu. But juicy berries offer far more than succulent taste and texture. They are a premier source of *anthocyanin,* an antioxidant with triple the power of vitamin C. This phytochemical is known to block cancer-causing cell damage and the effects of many age-related diseases. And when it comes to fighting age-related symptoms, the blueberry is king. Of all fruits and vegetables studied, blueberries have exhibited one of the highest antioxidant capacities, most likely due to their diverse range of phytochemicals, including anthocyanins.

Most of us have a limited season in which to enjoy berries at their prime; maybe that's why we love them so. But the tiny morsels are available year-round, both dried and frozen, offering the essence of their flavors for our cooking needs. Dried berries are preferred in some recipes. The water loss transforms their texture into a lasting chewy bite and concentrates their flavor so that it lingers longer.

What are you waiting for? Jump-start your day with Blueberry Upside-Down Clafouti, Blueberry Banana Muffins, Blackberry Mint Sorbet, or Warm Blueberry Compote. And in case you forgot, a bowl of plump, unadorned blueberries can work the same magic.

. . .

Another rising star is the regal strawberry. Strawberries stand toe to toe with oranges in terms of their vitamin C content. They are unsung heroes in bolstering immune strength, and they're right behind the blueberry in derailing age-related slumps in memory and balance.

An average strawberry contains about two hundred seeds, each of which is a concentrated source of yet another antioxidant, *ellagic acid*. The seeds contain more of this compound than the fruit's pulp. And the raspberry has even more. Ellagic acid has been found to promote healing and fight heart disease. It has also shown extraordinary promise in fighting cancer growth in a variety of studies. Explore the bold new flavors of these crimson kings in Strawberry Gelée and in Crispy Cornmeal Waffles with Warm Berry Syrup.

It's no wonder that the brilliant ruby-red of the cranberry is extracted for dyes or that its lively rustic contrast is a familiar fixture on a holiday tree. Cranberries have been around for eons and were in fact a key ingredient in the original "trail mix," known as *pemmican*. There are few foods as sour as the chubby cranberry; you would be hard-pressed to find a cranberry recipe, sweet or savory, that doesn't have a significant addition of sweetener to balance the berry's high acid content. Though you'd never know at first bite, the cranberry has a very sweet side. It is an excellent source of fiber, potassium, vitamin C, and, as is true for fruits and vegetables with vibrant color, it is packed with powerful phytochemicals.

Anyone who has ever had a urinary tract infection has heard another advisement, "Drink cranberry juice!" without knowing why. Well, we're still not certain, but mounting evidence supports a theory that the cranberry's unique combination of phytochemicals, including condensed tannins (or *proanthocyanidins*), creates an antiadhesion property that keeps bacteria from sticking where they might otherwise blossom into a full-blown infection. This may be beneficial throughout the body, including our mouth and gums. So don't limit your consumption to a dollop of relish come November. Crack open a bottle of the tangy garnet elixir for your next afternoon pick-me-up and slather Cranberry Spice Jam on your next muffin.

Crispy Vegetarian Spring Rolls with Shanghai Plum Sauce

Crispy and bursting with flavor, these spring rolls are baked, not fried. The piquant plum sauce can be made year-round since canned plums work well if fresh plums are not in season.

YIELD: 8 LARGE SPRING ROLLS AND 1 CUP SAUCE
PREPARATION TIME: 45 MINUTES

Spring Roll Filling:
1 tablespoon olive oil
1 medium finely chopped yellow onion
2 tablespoons minced garlic
2 tablespoons peeled, chopped fresh ginger
3 cups finely shredded green cabbage
½ cup grated carrot
½ cup chopped fresh cilantro, without stems
1 tablespoon low-sodium soy sauce
Salt to taste

Plum Sauce:
1 tablespoon olive oil
½ teaspoon yellow or black mustard seeds
1 tablespoon minced garlic
1 tablespoon peeled, chopped fresh ginger
¼ cup low-sodium soy sauce
2 tablespoons red wine vinegar
1 tablespoon sorghum syrup or dark honey
*¾ pound fresh Italian prune plums or 1 (16-ounce) can pitted plums,
    drained and rinsed of any syrup*

6 (12 x 17-inch) sheets phyllo dough, thawed overnight in the
  refrigerator
Olive oil cooking spray
2 tablespoons cornstarch dissolved in ½ cup water

Garnish:
Cilantro sprigs

Prepare spring roll filling: Heat olive oil in a large sauté pan over medium-high heat. Add onion and sauté until softened but not colored, 2 minutes. Add garlic and ginger and sauté 1 minute longer. Add cabbage and stir-fry until cabbage is softened, about 2 minutes.

Remove pan from heat. Add carrot, cilantro, and soy sauce. Stir until combined. Season with salt if desired. Transfer to a bowl to cool. (There should be about 2 cups of filling.)

Prepare plum sauce: Heat olive oil in a large sauté pan over medium-high heat. Add mustard seeds. Add garlic and ginger and sauté, stirring constantly, 30 seconds. Stir in soy sauce, vinegar, sorghum syrup, and plums. Simmer until slightly thickened, about 5 minutes. Transfer to the bowl of a food processor or a blender jar. Process or blend until smooth. Transfer to a small bowl and set aside.

Assemble spring rolls: Preheat oven to 400 degrees Fahrenheit. Lightly coat a 15 x 10-inch baking sheet with olive oil spray. Drain filling mixture to remove any excess liquid that may have accumulated during cooling. Filling should be very dry.

Carefully remove 3 sheets of phyllo dough from the package. Do not separate; keep the 3 sheets together. Cover remaining phyllo with a damp cloth to keep it from drying out. Cut the stack of 3 sheets into quarters with one crosswise and one lengthwise cut.

Arrange first quarter sheet (of 3 thicknesses) with the shortest side facing you. Spread ¼ cup of the filling along the short side, leaving a 1-inch border at each end. Fold the edges of each long side over the first inch of the filling and roll up the filling in the wrapper, rolling away from you. Seal the end of the roll with a light brushing of the cornstarch-water mixture. Transfer to the prepared baking sheet. Working quickly, repeat with remaining 3 sheets of phyllo dough and filling to make 4 more spring rolls.

Spray rolls with olive oil spray and bake immediately in hot oven for about 10 minutes, or until golden, turning over midway through baking to ensure even browning.

Garnish with cilantro sprigs. Serve with 1 tablespoon sauce per spring roll. Pass extra dipping sauce.

NOTE: Spring rolls may be assembled up to 2 hours ahead of baking time. Arrange rolls on the baking sheet so that they are not touching. Cover loosely with plastic wrap and refrigerate. They also may be assembled, separated with plastic, and frozen prior to baking. Add about 3 minutes to baking time.

Plum Factoid: Dried plums can be used as natural preservatives due to their ability to inhibit mold formation in baked goods.

Nutrient Analysis: per spring roll with 1 tablespoon plum sauce

CALORIES: 143 PROTEIN: 3 grams CARBOHYDRATES: 18 grams TOTAL FAT: 7 grams SATURATED FAT: 1 gram POLYUNSATURATED FAT: 1 gram MONOUNSATURATED FAT: 5 grams CHOLESTEROL: 0 mg FIBER: 2 grams (Soluble fiber 1 gram) SODIUM: 475 mgs

Savory Chicken Tagine with Slivered Dried Plums and Baby Artichokes

Though it's not prepared in the classic tagine vessel, this sumptuous stew has flavors that whisper "Morocco." Serve with a tomato or cucumber salad and steamed bulgur.

YIELD: 1½ QUARTS; 4 (1½ CUP) SERVINGS

PREPARATION TIME: 45 MINUTES

1 pound boneless, skinless chicken breasts
1 tablespoon olive oil
1 large chopped onion
3 cups fat-free chicken or vegetable broth
1 teaspoon crumbled saffron threads
¾ teaspoon salt
1½ medium (5 ounces) carrots, cut into ¼-inch dice
1½ teaspoons ground ginger

¾ teaspoon ground cinnamon

1 cup pitted dried plums, cut into slivers

9 ounces fresh artichoke hearts, quartered, or 1 (9-ounce) package
  frozen artichoke hearts, thawed and quartered lengthwise
  (see Note below)

½ cup chopped fresh cilantro, without stems

Cut chicken into 1-inch pieces. Heat oil in a 3-quart saucepan over medium-high heat until hot but not smoking. Add onion and sauté until softened, stirring to prevent browning.

Stir in broth, saffron, and salt and bring to a boil. Reduce heat to low. Add carrots and simmer, covered, about 2 minutes.

Add ginger, cinnamon, plums, and artichoke hearts and simmer until vegetables and fruits are nearly tender, about 2 minutes.

Add chicken pieces to stew and stir in cilantro. Simmer, uncovered, stirring occasionally, about 3 minutes or until chicken is just cooked.

NOTE: You may use a drained 9-ounce jar of water-packed artichoke hearts. Because they are already cooked, add them at the end, *after* the chicken is cooked.

Artichoke Factoid: A phytochemical in artichoke plants called *cynarin* is used by European doctors to lower elevated blood cholesterol. Unlike cholesterol-lowering drugs that can have toxic effects on the liver, cynarin is thought to *improve* liver function.

Nutrient Analysis: per 1½-cup serving

CALORIES: 335   PROTEIN: 34 grams   CARBS.: 39 grams   TOTAL FAT: 5 grams   SAT. FAT: 1 gram
POLY. FAT: 1 gram   MONO. FAT: 3 grams   CHOLES.: 39 mgs   FIBER: 7 grams (Sol. 2 grams)
SODIUM: 684 mgs

Crispy Cornmeal Waffles with Warm Berry Syrup

Sink your teeth through the crackly crust and taste the nutty flavors of this breakfast classic. The rich creamy syrup is loaded with chewy berries. The batter is a snap to make, though it's better if prepared the night before. If prepared the same day, allow the batter to set at least 30 minutes before baking.

YIELD: 12 (4-INCH) OR 6 (8-INCH) WAFFLES AND ABOUT 1½ CUPS SYRUP
PREPARATION TIME: 10 MINUTES

Waffles:
¾ cup unbleached all-purpose flour
1 cup stone-ground cornmeal
2 teaspoons baking powder
¼ teaspoon salt
¼ cup untoasted wheat germ
1 tablespoon ground flaxseed (see Note, page 32)
1 large egg
1 egg white
1¾ cups unflavored soymilk
¼ cup olive oil

Warm Berry Syrup:
1 cup fresh or frozen blueberries or raspberries
¾ cup sorghum syrup
1 teaspoon fresh lemon juice

Prepare waffles: Sift together flour, cornmeal, baking powder, and salt into a large mixing bowl. Stir in wheat germ and flaxseed. Whisk together egg, egg white, soymilk, and oil in another large bowl. Add flour mixture all at once and whisk just until combined. (There will be about 3 cups of batter.)

Preheat a waffle iron. Preheat oven to 275 degrees Fahrenheit. Spoon batter into waffle iron, using ¼ cup batter for each 4-inch-square waffle or ½ cup per 8-inch waffle. Spread batter evenly and cook according to manufacturer's instructions. (If batter is too thick to spread easily, thin with a little soymilk.) Transfer waffle to a baking sheet and keep warm, uncovered, in middle of the oven. Make more waffles with remaining batter in same manner. To ensure a crispy crust and creamy center, enjoy the waffles within 15 minutes of preparation. Serve waffles with Warm Berry Syrup.

Prepare Warm Berry Syrup: While waffles are cooking, in a small saucepan cook blueberries and sorghum syrup over low to medium heat until berries burst, about 3 minutes. Stir in lemon juice. The syrup keeps covered and refrigerated for 1 week. Reheat syrup before serving.

NOTE: Leftover waffles can be wrapped and frozen. Heat in a toaster on low setting for 1 minute for a quick and hearty breakfast.

Raspberry Factoid: Raspberries contain a phytochemical called *ellagic acid,* which is thought to inhibit the initiation stage of cancer cell growth caused by certain chemicals.

Nutrient Analysis: per 4-inch waffle with 1½ tablespoons syrup

CALORIES: 159   PROTEIN: 4 grams   CARBS.: 23 grams   TOTAL FAT: 6 grams   SAT. FAT: 1 gram
POLY. FAT: 1 gram   MONO. FAT: 4 grams   CHOLES.: 17 mgs   FIBER: 2 grams   SODIUM: 155 mgs

Warm Breakfast Grains with Dried Cherries and Toasted Pecans

In this unusual whole-grain dish, coarsely ground bulgur takes a sweet turn. A warm and satisfying breakfast, it also makes a delicious snack or dessert. This dish is loaded with fiber. Leftovers can be reheated.

YIELD: 3 CUPS; 6 (½-CUP) SERVINGS
PREPARATION TIME: 20 MINUTES

> 2 teaspoons olive oil
> 1 cup coarsely ground bulgur
> 1½ teaspoons peeled, finely minced fresh ginger
> 2¼ cups unflavored soymilk, plus extra for serving
> 2 tablespoons sorghum syrup or dark honey
> 1 (3-inch) cinnamon stick
> 1 cup chopped dried cherries
> ⅓ cup chopped toasted pecans or other nuts (see Note, page 31)

Heat oil in a 2-quart saucepan over medium heat. Add bulgur and ginger to pan and toast lightly, stirring occasionally, for about 3 minutes.

Carefully add soymilk and sorghum syrup and stir well. Add cinnamon stick and heat mixture over medium-high heat, but do not boil. Reduce heat to low and cover. Simmer, stirring occasionally, until most of the liquid has been absorbed but grains are still loose and creamy, about 13 minutes. Remove from heat and stir in cherries and nuts.

Serve warm, passing additional hot soymilk and cherries if desired.

NOTE: To toast nuts in the oven, preheat oven to 375 degrees Fahrenheit. Place the nuts on a baking sheet in a single layer and bake 5 to 8 minutes, or until fragrant. Stir nuts a few times during baking to ensure even browning. To toast on the stovetop, place nuts in small dry sauté pan over medium heat. Toast nuts, stirring occasionally, until fragrant and lightly browned, about 2 minutes. Set aside to cool.

Cherry Factoid: There are several different varieties of dried cherries on the market. One pound equals about 3½ cups.

Nutrient Analysis: per ½-cup serving
> CALORIES: 223   PROTEIN: 7 grams   CARBS.: 34 grams   TOTAL FAT: 7 grams   SAT. FAT: 1 gram
> POLY. FAT: 1 gram   MONO. FAT: 4 grams   CHOLES.: 0 mg   FIBER: 7 grams (Sol. 1 gram)
> SODIUM: 16 mgs

Blueberry Banana Muffins

Emerging health research has fueled a skyrocketing demand for this electric berry. One of the largest overseas importers of American blueberries is Japan. Their annual import of frozen blueberries recently topped 25 million pounds, an exponential increase from five years earlier. Savor the benefits of blueberries in moist, delicious muffins. They are loaded with fiber and freeze well, too.

YIELD: 12 MEDIUM MUFFINS
PREPARATION TIME: 25 MINUTES

> *1½ cups unprocessed wheat bran or oat bran*
> *¾ cup unbleached all-purpose flour*
> *¼ cup sorghum flour*

2 tablespoons ground flaxseed (see Note, below)
1¼ teaspoons baking soda
1 teaspoon ground cinnamon
⅛ teaspoon salt
¾ cup unflavored soymilk
½ cup sorghum syrup or dark honey
1 ripe medium banana, mashed with a fork
1 large egg
2 tablespoons olive oil
1 teaspoon pure vanilla extract
1 cup fresh or dried blueberries
½ cup pitted, chopped dates (optional)

Position a rack in the center of the oven and preheat oven to 400 degrees Fahrenheit. Lightly coat 12 (2¼ x 1½-inch) nonstick muffin cups with olive oil spray.

In a medium bowl, combine bran, flours, flaxseed, baking soda, cinnamon, and salt. Set aside. In another medium bowl or in a blender, combine soymilk, sorghum syrup, banana, egg, olive oil, and vanilla extract until smooth.

Make a well in the center of the dry ingredients and pour in ⅓ of the liquid mixture. Using a spoon, stir until smooth. Add remaining liquid mixture and stir just until combined. Add blueberries (and dates if desired); stir again, but do not overmix.

Spoon ¼ cup of batter into each prepared muffin cup. Bake about 14 minutes, or until the tops spring back when pressed gently in the centers. Do not overbake. Cool in the pan on a wire rack for 10 minutes before removing from the cups. Serve warm, or cool completely on the rack.

NOTE: Grind whole flaxseeds in a clean spice grinder to the consistency of cornmeal.

Blueberry Factoid: Color, not size, is an indicator of blueberry ripeness. Look for berries that are deep purple to blue-black.

Nutrient Analysis: per muffin

CALORIES: 253 PROTEIN: 6 grams CARBS.: 52 grams TOTAL FAT: 4 grams SAT. FAT: 1 gram
POLY. FAT: 1 gram MONO. FAT: 2 grams CHOLES.: 18 mgs FIBER: 5 grams (Sol. 1 gram)
SODIUM: 170 mgs

Cranberry Spice Jam

Not just for Thanksgiving, this jam is delicious year-round. Grab the peanut butter and whole-grain bread for a hearty breakfast sandwich.

YIELD: 4 CUPS; 32 (2-TABLESPOON) SERVINGS
PREPARATION TIME: 20 MINUTES

6 cups fresh cranberries or 2 (12-ounce) bags frozen cranberries
2 cups unsweetened Concord grape juice
1 cup sorghum syrup
1 tablespoon grated citrus peel (lemon, orange, or tangerine)
1 teaspoon ground ginger
½ teaspoon ground allspice
¼ teaspoon ground nutmeg

Wash cranberries and place in a heavy, 4-quart nonreactive saucepan. Add grape juice and sorghum syrup. Stir to combine.

Heat mixture over medium-high heat until the liquid is boiling and the cranberries start to pop. Reduce heat to low and simmer, stirring occasionally, for about 25 minutes or until berries are soft and juices thicken. Jam will continue to thicken as it cools.

Remove from heat. Stir in citrus peel and ground spices. Pour into clean sterilized jars. Cool and store in the refrigerator for up to 1 month.

Cranberry Factoid: Though cranberries are only found in the stores from October through December, they freeze well and will last until the next season. Freezing doesn't diminish their nutrient content either.

Nutrient Analysis: per 2-tablespoon serving

CALORIES: 50 PROTEIN: 0 gram CARBS.: 12 grams TOTAL FAT: 0 gram SAT. FAT: 0 gram POLY. FAT: 0 gram MONO. FAT: 0 gram CHOLES.: 0 mg FIBER: 1 gram SODIUM: 2 mgs

Blueberry Upside-Down Clafouti

Clafouti is a rustic French dessert topped by a layer of berries or fruit in a baking dish topped with a blanket of custardlike batter. An "accidental" discovery proved this clafouti to be gorgeous turned upside down! The result is a warm fruity concoction of chewy blueberries and dried plums floating atop a creamy pudding cake. The recipe works splendidly with other dried berries and fruits.

YIELD: 8-INCH ROUND; 9 SERVINGS
PREPARATION TIME: 40 MINUTES

1 cup pitted dried plums (6 ounces)
½ cup dried blueberries (3 ounces)
2 tablespoons stone-ground cornmeal
¾ cup unbleached all-purpose flour
½ teaspoon ground cinnamon
½ teaspoon salt
2 large eggs
1 large egg white
2 tablespoons olive oil

¼ cup sorghum syrup or dark honey
1½ cups unflavored soymilk
1 tablespoon pure vanilla extract

Position a rack in upper third of oven. Preheat oven to 350 degrees Fahrenheit. Lightly coat an 8-inch round layer cake pan with olive oil spray.

Cut dried plums into ¼-inch slivers and place in a small mixing bowl with the blueberries. Sprinkle berries and plums with cornmeal and toss to combine well. Transfer fruit to prepared baking pan. Arrange evenly to cover the bottom of the pan.

Combine flour, cinnamon, and salt in a medium mixing bowl, making a well in the center. In another medium mixing bowl, whisk together eggs, egg white, olive oil, sorghum syrup, soymilk, and vanilla.

Pour ⅓ of the egg mixture over dry ingredients and whisk until smooth. Add remaining egg mixture and stir just to combine. Do not overbeat.

Carefully pour batter over the fruit (the fruit may float to the top) and bake in upper third of the oven about 40 minutes or until egg mixture puffs and sets in the center.

Transfer clafouti to a rack to cool for 30 minutes. Invert onto a serving platter. Serve clafouti warm or at room temperature.

Blueberry Factoid: Studies have shown that the content of antioxidant phytochemicals in blueberries increases with the maturity of the berry.

Nutrient Analysis: per serving

CALORIES: 209   PROTEIN: 5 grams   CARBS.: 38 grams   TOTAL FAT: 5 grams   SAT. FAT: 1 gram
POLY. FAT: 1 gram   MONO. FAT: 3 grams   CHOLES.: 34 mgs   FIBER: 3 grams (Sol. 1 gram)
SODIUM: 39 mgs

Strawberry Gelée

The essence of fully ripened berries flavors this light and refreshing treat. Served in an elegant stemmed glass with fresh berries, it's a showstopper. It's also a great snack and an inventive way to use an excess of fresh berries. To retain optimal levels of ellagic acid and its antiaging benefits, do not strain the seeds from the berry purée. Serve with additional fresh or dried berries.

YIELD: 3 CUPS; 4 (¾-CUP) SERVINGS
PREPARATION TIME: 20 MINUTES PLUS 2 HOURS SETTING TIME

> 3 cups hulled fresh strawberries or 1 (12-ounce) bag frozen strawberries
> ⅓ cup sorghum syrup or dark honey
> 1 tablespoon fresh lime juice
> ¼ teaspoon pure vanilla extract
> ⅛ teaspoon ground ginger
> 1 teaspoon finely chopped fresh mint, without stems
> ½ cup cold water
> 1 (¼-ounce) envelope unflavored gelatin powder
> ¾ cup boiling water

Puree strawberries in a food processor or blender. Add sorghum syrup, lime juice, vanilla, ginger, and mint.

Pour cold water into a 1-quart nonreactive mixing bowl. Sprinkle gelatin over water and allow to soften for about 3 minutes. Whisk in boiling water until dissolved. Allow to cool to room temperature, about 10 minutes. (Do not wait too long or gelatin will solidify.) Stir in berry purée and taste for sweetness. Add additional 1 tablespoon sorghum syrup if berries aren't sweet enough.

Pour mixture into four serving bowls and refrigerate until set, about 2 hours. Refrigerate up to 2 days.

Strawberry Factoid: The size of a strawberry does not determine its flavor. All strawberries, large or small, can be equally delicious if grown and harvested properly and if they are ripe when consumed.

Nutrient Analysis: per ¾-cup serving

CALORIES: 118   PROTEIN: 2 grams   CARBS.: 30 grams   TOTAL FAT: 0 gram   SAT. FAT: 0 gram   POLY. FAT: 0 gram   MONO. FAT: 0 gram   CHOLES.: 0 mg   FIBER: 2 grams   SODIUM: 4 mgs

Warm Blueberry Compote

A hint of cloves adds depth to this vibrantly colored compote with a rich texture and full flavor. It will be well received, whether it is used to top pancakes, sorbet, or fresh fruit. It is also a simple way to enhance a steaming bowl of hot cereal. Savor its sweetest attribute: The blueberry ranks the highest in antioxidant activity of forty other fruits and vegetables.

YIELD: 2 CUPS; 4 (½-CUP) SERVINGS
PREPARATION TIME: 10 MINUTES

> *2 cups fresh or frozen blueberries*
> *1 tablespoon fresh lemon juice*
> *3 tablespoons sorghum syrup or dark honey*
> *1 teaspoon pure vanilla extract*
> *1 teaspoon grated lemon peel*
> *Pinch ground cloves*

Combine all ingredients in a 1-quart saucepan and bring to a boil over medium heat. Cover and simmer until juices are slightly thickened, about 5 minutes. Frozen berries may take slightly longer to thicken.

Remove from heat and serve.

Blueberry Factoid: The antioxidants found in blueberries fight aging and can reduce the risk of heart disease and some cancers.

Nutrient Analysis: per ½-cup serving
>   CALORIES: 66 PROTEIN: 1 gram CARBS.: 16 grams TOTAL FAT: 0 gram SAT. FAT: 0 gram
>   POLY. FAT: 0 gram MONO. FAT: 0 gram CHOLES.: 0 mg FIBER: 1 gram SODIUM: 4 mgs

Blackberry Mint Sorbet

The rich stunning color of this creamy, luscious dessert disguises the fact that it is refreshingly light. Serve with fresh berries or fruit.

>   YIELD: 2 CUPS; 4 (½-CUP) SERVINGS
>   PREPARATION TIME: 45 MINUTES

>   *¼ cup sorghum syrup or dark honey*
>   *¼ cup cassis (black currant) liqueur*
>   *¼ cup fresh mint leaves, without stems*
>   *2¼ cups fresh blackberries or 1 (16-ounce) bag frozen unsweetened*
>   *blackberries, thawed*

Combine sorghum syrup, liqueur, and mint leaves in a small heavy nonreactive saucepan over low heat. Cook until mixture is hot but not boiling. Remove from heat; cool. Strain to remove the mint.

Place berries in a food processor or a blender. Add cooled syrup and process until smooth.

Chill in the refrigerator until very cold. Freeze mixture in an ice-cream maker according to manufacturer's instructions.

Serve with additional berries if desired.

NOTE: To retain optimal levels of ellagic acid and its antiaging benefits, do not strain the seeds from the berry purée.

Blackberry Factoid: Not all blackberries are actually black. There are over one thousand kinds of blackberries, which range in color from black to burgundy and even to yellowish white.

Nutrient Analysis: per ½-cup serving

CALORIES: 178   PROTEIN: 3 grams   CARBS.: 38 grams   TOTAL FAT: 0 gram   SAT. FAT: 0 mg

POLY. FAT: 0 gram   MONO. FAT: 0 gram   CHOLES.: 0 mg   FIBER: 2 grams   SODIUM: 5 mgs

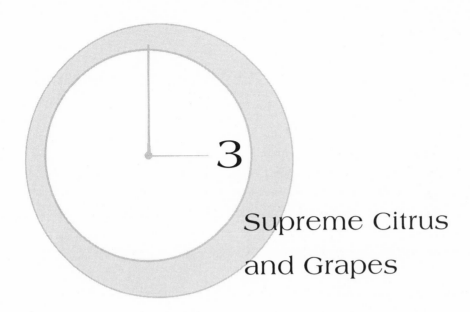

3

Supreme Citrus
and Grapes

What do citrus and grapes have in common? Aside from incredible flavor, the common denominator isn't apparent. But the mosaic of their vibrant colors conceals astonishing antiaging capacity and culinary utility.

CITRUS

Citrus fruits sing to our senses. Their radiant colors, bracing scents, and lush flavors make us pucker and smile. Drinking citrus is like sipping sunshine. Whether enjoyed as sweet pulpy nectar in the frosty glass we raise upon waking or as a warm and tangy dessert that heralds the end of our day, citrus is a culinary chameleon. Its guises are endless, whether savored in the chewiness of sweet candied peel, the astringency of tart vinaigrette, or the simple squeeze of freshness that punctuates a steaming cup of tea. Universally appealing, citrus also contains some amazing healing compounds that give a new ring to its zing.

The vibrant outer peels of lemons, limes, and their citrus partners contain oil glands like our own skin. A compound produced in these glands, called *limonene,* creates the explosion of citrus scent that erupts when a lemon peel is grated, but limonene does much more than just smell good. It is an antiaging gold mine. Here's why: Our bodies possess an important detoxifying enzyme, *glutathione transferase,* which fights cancer. Limonene appears to increase its benevolent activity. Its effects are thought to inhibit a variety of cancers by turning off a signal that otherwise allows carcinogenic cells to proliferate. Additional compounds found in citrus peel, *coumarin, kaempherol,* and *luteolin,* elicit similar responses. Scientists are also studying the potential of a component specific to lemon oil. They hope that its antioxidant capacity is also effective externally as an age retardant for skin.

The power of citrus doesn't stop at the peel. The juice boasts as much utility as it does flavor. Hesperidin, naringin, and quercetin are phytochemicals in citrus juice called *flavonoids.* It seems their brawn not only lowers the liver's production of cholesterol but also inhibits blood clot formation *and* boosts the bang of vitamin C, making it an even more effective scavenger of free radicals.

Citrus fruits contain additional phytochemicals and vitamins called *carotenoids,* such as beta-carotene, lycopene (especially in pink grapefruit), lutein, zeaxanthin, and beta-cryptoxanthin. A high intake of these substances has been associated with lower incidence of age-related macular degeneration (ARMD), the leading and perhaps most preventable cause of vision loss among the aged.

Citrus is also loaded with soluble fiber. The primary form, pectin, binds and consequently dilutes carcinogenic substances in the intestinal tract, lowers cholesterol, and helps regulate glucose levels.

Fill your juice glass to the rim and savor the flavors of citrus throughout the day. Lemon Tahini Sauce, Preserved Lemons, Stop the Clock! Cranberry-Grape Juice, and Sweet and Spicy Orange Salad are just a few of the ways you can reap more benefits from the popular citrus family.

GRAPES

Another luminary of antiaging fruits is the intensely hued purple grape. Though there are many varieties, most of us are familiar with the Concord-type purple grape. Occasionally, juicy purple grapes make their way to our produce aisles, but they're not nearly as popular for snacking as crisp red and green table grapes, probably because they have seeds. And although we may not favor grape seeds, not everyone is tossing them. Purple grape seeds are loaded with antioxidants, and many commercial juice companies are extracting this goodness and pouring them back in the juice for a supercharged punch.

Because of their strong association with juice and jelly, we generally turn to the unctuous sweetness of purple grapes at breakfast time. But here are enticing reasons to indulge *throughout* the day:

- In terms of antioxidant power, purple grapes are tops among a variety of fruits and vegetables at battling free radicals.
- Recent studies reveal that regular consumption of purple grape juice may promote significant cardiovascular benefits, including a decreased tendency for blood platelets to clot, reduced cholesterol levels, and increased levels of vitamin E, a key antioxidant.

If you're still not convinced, Purple Grape Jelly and PB&J Granola Bars are two more sumptuous reasons to enjoy purple grapes at breakfast time and beyond.

Falling not so far from the purple grapevine is a noble relative, the red wine grape. The course of culinary history was altered in the 1970s with the unveiling of the French paradox. The results of that research revealed that drinking red wine had cardioprotective benefits and gave us another welcome reason to indulge in this healthful libation. But researchers have continued to stir up clues that substantiate this theory, and then some.

The hidden gems in red grape juice and its fermented counterpart, wine, play a vital role in the fight against aging, thanks to phytochemicals called flavonoids. Resveratrol, ellagic acid, anthocyanins, and quercetin are just a few of them, and their impact is profound.

Though most scientists believe that polyphenols in red wine are responsible for lowering blood cholesterol, the mechanism isn't clear. Recent studies examined the effect of red wine's polyphenols on *endothelin-1,* a blood protein and a potent blood vessel constrictor. Too much endothelin-1 is thought to contribute to blockage in constricted arteries, increasing the risk of a heart attack. Red wine, as opposed to white or rosé wine, or even red grape juice, is effective at reducing blood levels of endothelin-1. This suggests that something in the wine-making process changes the pigment's properties. Earlier evidence that red wine dilates blood vessels and stops red blood cells from clumping may be an independent benefit or a consequence of suppressed endothelin-1 production.

Protection from heart disease isn't the only benefit of red wine's flavonoids. Their antioxidant properties are believed to fight against age-related mental decline. They also appear to minimize inflammation and discomfort of painful diseases such as arthritis. Like other antioxidants, they fight to keep our inveterate contingent of free radicals under control. Red wine is well endowed with resveratrol, and its concentration relates proportionately to the length of time the grape skins are present during the fermentation process in wine making. That's why the levels are significantly higher in red wine than in white wine. In some studies, this flavonoid also has shown promise in slowing the growth of cancer.

It is premature to recommend increased consumption of red wine. It is still an alcoholic beverage, and moderation is advised because of other potential health risks. One concern is resveratrol's structure, which is similar to that of the hormone estrogen. The potential benefits of this plant hormone could backfire if consumed in excessive amounts, resulting in promotion of hormonally related cancers, such as breast or prostate cancer.

Like other phytochemicals, we do know that they appear to be most beneficial when consumed in their natural form and in moderation from a variety of other whole-food sources. The synergy of their collective powers seems to provide the optimal benefit.

Raise your glass and relish the gifts that red wine grapes offer in Mulled Red Wine. Enjoy them as nature intended.

Sweet and Spicy Orange Salad

Hardly a ho-hum fruit salad, this exotic dish drizzles pungently spiced vinaigrette over plump orange slices. It's luscious chilled or at room temperature.

YIELD: 1 QUART; 8 (½-CUP) SERVINGS
PREPARATION TIME: 45 MINUTES

10 large navel oranges
3 tablespoons extra-virgin olive oil
½ teaspoon salt
1 teaspoon ground cinnamon

1 teaspoon ground coriander

1 teaspoon ground cumin

1½ teaspoons minced garlic

1 tablespoon chopped fresh cilantro, without stems

1 tablespoon chopped fresh Italian parsley, without stems

Scrub oranges with an abrasive sponge to remove any surface impurities. Rinse thoroughly; dry well.

Remove peel from two of the oranges with a zester or citrus grater. Set aside. (Peel from other oranges may be removed and reserved for another use.) Remove the peel and pith from all of the oranges. Slice oranges crosswise into ½-inch-thick rounds. Place slices in a mixing bowl.

Combine remaining ingredients in another bowl. Pour dressing over oranges and toss carefully.

Orange Factoid: Most of the vitamin C in oranges is found in the peel (53 percent), while lesser amounts are found in the juice (23 percent) and in the pulp (21 percent).

Nutrient Analysis: per ½-cup serving

CALORIES: 136   PROTEIN: 2 grams   CARBS.: 26 grams   TOTAL FAT: 5 grams   SAT. FAT: 0 gram
POLY. FAT: 0 gram   MONO. FAT: 4 grams   CHOLES.: 0 mg   FIBER: 1 gram   SODIUM: 1 mg

Lemon Tahini Sauce

Creamy, tangy, garlicky, and vibrantly yellow, this sauce is the perfect condiment to liven up a simple sandwich or a moist fish filet. The best part of all is that it takes just minutes to prepare.

YIELD: 1 CUP; 16 (1-TABLESPOON) SERVINGS
PREPARATION TIME: 5 MINUTES

½ cup tahini (see Note below)
⅓ cup plus 1 tablespoon fresh lemon juice
1½ teaspoons ground cumin
1 teaspoon ground turmeric
2 minced garlic cloves
1 tablespoon low-sodium soy sauce
4 tablespoons warm water
2 teaspoons minced Preserved Lemon peel (page 48) or grated fresh
* lemon peel*
¼ cup minced fresh cilantro, without stems

Combine tahini, lemon juice, cumin, turmeric, garlic, and soy sauce in the bowl of a food processor or blender; process or blend until smooth.

Thin mixture by adding water, 1 tablespoon at a time, until consistency of thick cream.

Pour sauce into a small nonreactive mixing bowl. Stir in lemon peel and cilantro until combined.

> **NOTE:** Tahini is a paste made from ground sesame seeds. It can be found in Middle Eastern markets or in the ethnic section of most supermarkets. It should be refrigerated after opening.

Lemon Factoids: To obtain the most juice from a fresh lemon, roll it around on a hard surface. This technique breaks down the pulp and membranes of the fruit, allowing for easier flow of juice once it is cut.

The average lemon weighs about 5 ounces and yields about 1 tablespoon of grated peel and 3 tablespoons of juice.

Nutrient Analysis: per 1-tablespoon serving

CALORIES: 50   PROTEIN: 2 grams   CARBS.: 3 grams   TOTAL FAT: 4 grams   SAT. FAT: 1 gram
POLY. FAT: 2 grams   MONO. FAT: 2 grams   CHOLES.: 0 mg   FIBER: 1 gram   SODIUM: 17 mgs

Preserved Lemons*

Preserved lemons are a staple in Moroccan cuisine. Their unique flavor and texture add a distinctive taste to salads and stews. Although easy to prepare, the lemons must cure for one month before using.

YIELD: 1 QUART
PREPARATION TIME: 20 MINUTES PLUS ONE MONTH CURING TIME

> *12 medium lemons*
> *¾ cup coarse salt (kosher or coarse sea salt)*
> *6 coriander seeds*
> *6 black peppercorns*
> *1 cinnamon stick*
> *4 whole cloves*

Scrub the lemons with an abrasive sponge to remove any surface impurities. Rinse thoroughly; dry well. Quarter eight of the lemons lengthwise and place in a medium non-reactive mixing bowl. Pour salt over lemons and toss well.

---

*For those not inclined to preserve their own lemons, see Shopping Sources on pages 235–237 for stores that sell this product.

Place half of the quartered lemons in a clean 1-quart jar. Add spices. Add remaining lemon halves, pressing down if necessary to ensure fit.

Juice the remaining four lemons. Add enough juice to cover the quartered lemons by ½ inch. If the lemons are not submerged in juice, add cool water to cover them. The lemons must be completely submerged in the salted lemon juice.

Allow lemons to cure in a cool dry place for 30 days. Invert jar daily if possible. Store the lemons in the refrigerator for up to 1 year.

To use, remove desired amount of lemon from the jar with clean metal tongs. Quickly rinse the lemon under running water, removing excess salt and discarding seeds. Chop as desired.

Preserved Lemon Factoid: For a new twist, substitute Preserved Lemon peel in your favorite recipes that call for an equivalent amount of fresh lemon peel. Polenta, risotto, and vinaigrettes will take on an exotic flavor.

Nutrient Analysis: per 1 teaspoon
CALORIES: 1   PROTEIN: 0 gram   CARBS.: 0 gram   TOTAL FAT: 0 gram   SAT. FAT: 0 gram
POLY. FAT: 0 gram   MONO. FAT: 0 gram   CHOLES.: 0 mg   FIBER: 0 gram   SODIUM: 299 mgs

Stop the Clock! Cranberry-Grape Juice

This refreshing juice provides a convenient pick-me-up and an antiaging triple whammy with cranberries, purple grapes, and citrus limonenes. The best part of all is that there is no added sweetener.

YIELD: 1 QUART; 8 (½-CUP) SERVINGS
PREPARATION TIME: 15 MINUTES

3 cups fresh cranberries or 1 (12-ounce) bag frozen cranberries
1 quart unsweetened Concord grape juice
Pinch salt
1 teaspoon grated citrus peel (lemon, lime, orange, or tangerine)

Rinse cranberries and transfer them to a 2-quart nonreactive saucepan. Add juice, salt, and citrus peel. Bring juice to a boil, reduce heat to medium, and simmer until the cranberries burst, about 10 minutes.

Strain the juice (without pressing cranberries) through a cheesecloth-lined sieve.

Chill juice and serve cold. (Cooked cranberries retain their flavor and can be reserved for another use such as Cranberry Spice Jam [page 33].)

Purple Grape Factoid: Shop carefully for purple grape juice, as some purple juices are blended with white grape juice. Purple grapes have plenty of natural sweetness; be sure the label says "unsweetened."

Nutrient Analysis: per ½-cup serving

CALORIES: 81   PROTEIN: 1 gram   CARBS.: 21 grams   TOTAL FAT: 0 gram   SAT. FAT: 0 gram
POLY. FAT: 0 gram   MONO. FAT: 0 gram   CHOLES.: 0 mg   FIBER: 1 gram   SODIUM: 4 mgs

Purple Grape Jelly

Most commercial purple grape jams and jellies use sugar as a primary ingredient. This recipe is easy, economical, and relies on the natural sweetness of the grapes and a small amount of sorghum syrup. Gelatin is used as a thickener, because most pectin products contain sugar. (Gelatin is also much cheaper.) This recipe is bursting with antioxidants. The jelly keeps for about a month, refrigerated—unless you make a few batches of PB&J Granola Bars (page 50)!

YIELD: 3½ CUPS; 26 (2-TABLESPOON) SERVINGS
PREPARATION TIME: 15 MINUTES

3 cups unsweetened Concord grape juice
2 tablespoons fresh lime juice
¼ cup sorghum syrup
2 (¼-ounce) envelopes unflavored gelatin powder

Pour juices and sorghum syrup into a 2-quart nonreactive saucepan. Sprinkle gelatin over juices and allow to soften for 2 minutes. Stir well. Bring juice mixture to a full rolling boil to dissolve gelatin. Remove from heat. Stir again. Pour into a clean, sterilized, 1-quart jar or 2 pint-size jars. Allow to cool slightly and seal. Cool and refrigerate for up to 1 month.

Purple Grape Factoid: The phytochemicals in purple grape juice are thought to reduce the "stickiness" of platelets in our blood. Platelet stickiness contributes to clotting, which can result in heart attack or stroke.

Nutrient Analysis: per 2-tablespoon serving

CALORIES: 29   PROTEIN: 1 gram   CARBS.: 7 grams   TOTAL FAT: 0 gram   SAT. FAT: 0 gram
POLY. FAT: 0 gram   MONO. FAT: 0 gram   CHOLES.: 0 mg   FIBER: 0 gram   SODIUM: 2 mgs

PB&J Granola Bars

An old favorite takes on a new form in chewy granola bars enriched with chunky peanut butter and bursts of grape jam. Perfect for a lunch box, the granola bars make a great snack for kids of all ages. Sugar-free jams and fruit spreads substitute well for grape jam or jelly. Cranberry Spice Jam is another tangy alternative.

YIELD: 32 BARS
PREPARATION TIME: 45 MINUTES

4½ cups old-fashioned rolled oats
¾ cup unbleached all-purpose flour
¼ cup sorghum flour
1 teaspoon baking soda
⅔ cup chunky natural peanut butter
½ cup sorghum syrup

½ cup vanilla soymilk
2 tablespoons olive oil
1 tablespoon pure vanilla extract
1 cup Concord grape jam or jelly

Preheat oven to 325 degrees Fahrenheit. Lightly coat a 13 x 9-inch baking pan with olive oil spray.

Combine all the ingredients except the jam in a large mixing bowl; mix well. Gently press half of the oat mixture into the prepared pan. Spread jam evenly over the oat mixture. Crumble remaining oat mixture evenly over the jam layer. Press down with palm of your hand to flatten slightly.

Bake about 25 minutes, or until golden brown. Let cool 10 minutes and cut into bars. Let bars cool completely in pan before removing or serving.

Grape Factoid: In comparison to all plants, grapes have the highest content of *resveratrol.* This phenolic compound, which is concentrated in their skins, has exhibited promising antioxidant effects in the areas of cardiovascular and cancer research.

Nutrient Analysis: per bar

CALORIES: 144 PROTEIN: 4 grams CARBS.: 23 grams TOTAL FAT: 4 grams SAT. FAT: 1 gram
POLY. FAT: 1 gram MONO. FAT: 2 grams CHOLES.: 0 mg FIBER: 3 grams (Sol. 1 gram)
SODIUM: 71 mgs

Mulled Red Wine

Mulled wine is a medieval libation that has never lost its popularity. There's no need to use an expensive wine, but be sure to choose a dry red wine with deep, full flavor. Removing the whole spices is easy and allows the wine to retain its clarity. Instead of sugar syrup, Concord grape juice and a small amount of sorghum syrup are used as sweeteners. For a nonalcoholic twist, try cranberry juice instead of red wine.

YIELD: 3 CUPS; 6 (½-CUP) SERVINGS
PREPARATION TIME: 10 MINUTES

1 lemon
1 orange
12 whole cloves
2 (3-inch) cinnamon sticks
4 (¼-inch) slices peeled fresh ginger
⅛ teaspoon ground nutmeg
¾ cup unsweetened Concord grape juice
¼ cup sorghum syrup
1 (750-ml) bottle medium- to full-bodied red wine

Garnish:
6 (3-inch) cinnamon sticks

Clean lemon and orange with an abrasive sponge to remove impurities. Rinse well. Remove peels with a vegetable peeler in large strips. Reserve whole fruits for another use.

Combine citrus peel, spices, and grape juice in a 2-quart nonreactive saucepan. Bring to a boil, reduce heat to low, and simmer 5 minutes. Remove from heat and cool completely, allowing flavors to infuse.

Add sorghum syrup and wine to the saucepan. Heat mixture over medium heat until hot, but do not boil. Strain to remove the spices. Pour into glasses or mugs and garnish with a cinnamon stick.

Red Wine Grape Factoid: Studies comparing grape varieties have shown that reds have higher contents of key phytochemicals (flavonoids, phenols) in comparison with whites.

Nutrient Analysis: per ½-cup serving

CALORIES: 156   PROTEIN: 1 gram   CARBS.: 18 grams   TOTAL FAT: 0 gram   SAT. FAT: 0 gram
POLY. FAT: 0 gram   MONO. FAT: 0 gram   CHOLES.: 0 mg   FIBER: 0 gram   SODIUM: 11 mgs

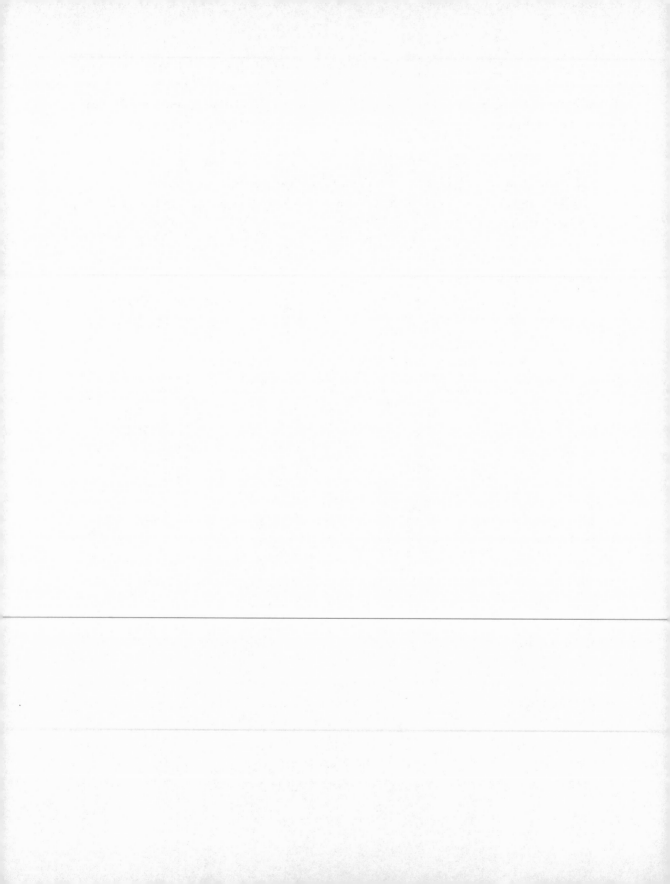

4 Time-Honored Tomatoes

The seductive scent of a plump ripe tomato beckons us to take a bite. Juicy tomatoes taste like summer; no enhancement is required. From Kashmir to Guadalajara, tomatoes have been savored for centuries. Imagine people from all over the world standing over a sink with a salt shaker in one hand and a juicy tomato in the other. It's a common thread. We can give thanks to sixteenth-century European explorers who returned from Peru with tomatoes. Five centuries later, this global tomato has not lost its appeal. Whether hot and spicy in a Bengali curry or cool and refreshing in an icy gazpacho, tomatoes are a versatile and much-loved ingredient.

How do tomatoes fit into the antiaging picture? The secret is *lycopene,* a plant pigment that brings the blush of red to the tomato (green and orange tomatoes have lesser amounts). Considered a vegetable by most, tomatoes are actually the fruit of a plant from the Lycopersicon family, hence the name *lycopene.* Smaller amounts of this pigment are found in other fruits, such as watermelon, pink grapefruit, and guavas.

Lycopene is a carotenoid, and, like the beta-carotene found in carrots, it is a powerful antioxidant. Although beta-carotene may be converted into vitamin A, lycopene cannot. On the other hand, it is capable of slowing or halting oxidative processes that may prevent or deter the onset of many diseases associated with aging. In recent studies, men and women who had heart attacks had lower tissue levels of lycopene than those with healthy hearts. More recent research indicates that people with low lycopene levels showed significant evidence of carotid artery thickening, a prime indicator of cardiovascular disease. Better heart health isn't the only reason to eat tomatoes. Tomato-Lentil Soup, Tomato Jam with Lemon and Basil, and Southwestern Barbecue Sauce with Chipotle Chiles are a few more delicious reasons.

Lycopene can also slash the odds of prostate and other cancers. Dr. David Heber of UCLA, a leading authority on nutrition and cancer believes, ". . . we have more evidence that lycopene may be beneficial to health than for any other phytochemical. I recommend at least five servings per week to obtain its full benefits. And since lycopene is liberated from tomato flesh during cooking, this is one example where heating *improves* the nutritional quality of food." Dr. Heber believes that ". . . a high consumption of tomato products can reduce the risk of prostate cancer by nearly 40 percent." It has also shown a decreased risk for lung and stomach cancers. It's easy to increase your intake when you add Icy Gazpacho with Fresh Lime and Corn Tortilla Spikes, Tomato-Ginger Bisque, or Roasted Tomato Curry with Gingered Garbanzo Beans and Baby Spinach to your menu.

Pasta sauce can keep your face from wrinkling. Well, sort of. In the 1930s, peasant women in Hungary applied tomato slices to their cheeks to reduce irritations from working in the fields. A fellow countrywoman, Madame Ella Baché, subsequently developed a skin cream called *Crème Tomate* and catalyzed a revolution in cosmetics based on natural fruit acids to refine the texture of skin. But tomatoes also work from the inside.

The dreaded signs of sagging and wrinkling are for most of us an inevitable part of growing older. Damage from the sun's ultraviolet (UV) rays exponentially increases and sometimes accelerates the process. Lycopene seems to protect against harmful ultraviolet rays. A Tufts study of sixty-something women revealed that skin levels of lycopene were rapidly depleted after UV exposure, suggesting that lycopene reserves were exhausted by free radicals.

The damaging effects of the sun's harmful rays are not limited to the skin; they can also harm our vision by damaging the macula, the part of the retina located at the back of the eye. The macula distinguishes fine detail in our central field of vision. Sometimes small blood vessels of the eye become narrowed and hardened, which blocks blood flow to the macula, causing its degeneration. Blurred central vision follows. Ultraviolet rays from the sun can damage the retina, promoting macular degeneration. The natural yellow color of the macula is due to the presence of carotenoids, lutein, and zeaxanthin. A diet rich in antioxidants, including lycopene, may help stave off degeneration of the macula.

The lycopene in tomatoes is concentrated during the cooking process because of the water loss that occurs. Tomato paste and ketchup are the richest sources. Because lycopene is fat-soluble, cooking tomatoes with a small amount of oil will further increase lycopene absorption by the body. Full of fiber and vitamin C, tomatoes are a winning first step toward living a healthier life. Find a cure in your cupboard and boost your vitality with Smoky Tomato Stew with Country Bread and Cannellini Beans, and Savory Moussaka with Pumate Béchamel.

Tomato-Lentil Soup

A traditional Indian soup, this is also known as *rasa,* or tomato dal. A thicker version, using less broth, is often served with rice as a main dish. This richly perfumed classic can be made ahead and will keep well for 2 days if refrigerated. It can also be frozen for up to 1 month.

YIELD: 1¼ QUARTS; 6 (¾-CUP) SERVINGS
PREPARATION TIME: 45 MINUTES

½ cup dry yellow lentils
4 cups fat-free chicken or vegetable broth
1 tablespoon olive oil
1½ teaspoons black or yellow mustard seeds
1 pound peeled, seeded, chopped plum tomatoes
    (see Note, page 195)
3 tablespoons peeled, finely chopped fresh ginger
1 minced garlic clove
1 teaspoon ground coriander
1 teaspoon ground cumin

1 teaspoon ground turmeric
Pinch cinnamon
¼ cup chopped fresh cilantro, without stems
Salt to taste

Wash lentils and drain well in a sieve. Combine lentils and 1½ cups of the broth in a 2-quart saucepan. Bring to a boil, reduce heat, and simmer lentils over low heat until they are tender but still retain their shape (about 30 minutes).

Meanwhile, heat olive oil in a heavy 4-quart saucepan over medium-high heat until hot but not smoking. Add mustard seeds and cook, stirring, until seeds just begin to pop. Carefully add tomatoes, ginger, garlic, and spices. Simmer until tomatoes are softened and spices are fragrant, about 4 minutes. Add 1½ cups of the broth and bring to a boil. Reduce heat and simmer, stirring occasionally, for about 4 minutes.

Carefully transfer the tomato-ginger mixture to the bowl of a food processor or a blender jar. Process or blend until smooth. Return to saucepan and add cooked lentils and the remaining 1 cup of chicken broth, stirring to incorporate. Bring soup to a boil, stirring occasionally. Stir in cilantro. Season with salt.

Tomato Factoid: Tomatine, a substance found in tomato leaves and unripened tomatoes, is known to heal certain fungal diseases of the skin.

Nutrient Analysis: per ¾-cup serving

CALORIES: 125   PROTEIN: 10 grams   CARBS.: 14 grams   TOTAL FAT: 3 grams   SAT. FAT: 0 gram

POLY. FAT: 0 gram   MONO. FAT: 2 grams   CHOLES.: 0 mg   FIBER: 6 grams (Sol. 1 gram)

SODIUM: 123 mgs

Icy Gazpacho with Fresh Lime and Corn Tortilla Spikes

The southern region of Spain is the birthplace of this refreshing summer favorite. The sweetness of plump ripened tomatoes mingles with the fresh flavors of garden vegetables, cilantro, and a hint of balsamic vinegar. Serve chilled with crunchy garlic bread or fresh croutons.

YIELD: 1½ QUARTS; 4 (1½-CUP) SERVINGS
PREPARATION TIME: 1 HOUR

4 corn tortillas, cut into ¼-inch-wide strips
1 large red bell pepper
2 large peeled tomatoes or 6 peeled plum tomatoes (about 1 pound)
1 large peeled, seeded cucumber, halved lengthwise
½ medium yellow onion
1 cup tomato juice
½ cup chopped fresh cilantro, without stems
¼ cup balsamic vinegar
2 tablespoons fresh lime juice
Salt and pepper to taste

Preheat oven to 350 degrees Fahrenheit. Line a 15 x 10-inch baking sheet with foil. Lightly coat foil with olive oil spray and arrange tortilla strips in a single layer. Bake about 8 minutes, or until crisp and golden, turning once. Set aside.

Roast the whole red pepper under a broiler or over a gas flame, turning occasionally, until the skin blisters and chars all over. Place in a bowl, cover with a lid, and allow it to steam to loosen the skin, or place in a paper bag and fold ends to enclose. Carefully peel away the skin and remove the seeds. Cut the pepper into medium dice and set aside.

Cut half of the tomatoes, half of the cucumber, and half of the onion into 1-inch pieces and transfer to the bowl of a food processor or a blender jar. Add the roasted bell pepper and puree. Transfer mixture to a medium mixing bowl. Add tomato juice, cilantro, and vinegar.

Seed the remaining tomato. Cut remaining tomato, cucumber, and onion into medium dice and add to the soup. Refrigerate until chilled.

Add lime juice before serving and season with salt and pepper. Serve well chilled, garnished with corn tortilla spikes. For a less chunky gazpacho, thin with additional tomato juice.

Tomato Factoid: Juicing tomatoes that haven't been cooked results in separation of the juice due to an enzyme that is activated when tomatoes are cut or crushed. Cooking the tomatoes first inactivates the enzyme, and the juiced tomatoes won't separate.

Nutrient Analysis: per 1½-cup serving

CALORIES: 119 PROTEIN: 4 grams CARBS.: 28 grams TOTAL FAT: 1 gram SAT. FAT: 0 gram
POLY. FAT: 0 gram MONO. FAT: 1 gram CHOLES.: 0 mg FIBER: 5 grams SODIUM: 61 mgs

Tomato-Ginger Bisque

America's all-time favorite soup is spiced with ginger to give it an exotic accent. A steaming bowl served with crusty bread provides the ultimate meal of simple comfort food. Ginger is also an excellent digestive. If you are endowed with an abundant tomato harvest, make extra batches of this recipe and freeze to enjoy later.

YIELD: 1 QUART; 4 (1-CUP) SERVINGS
PREPARATION TIME: 45 MINUTES

1 tablespoon olive oil
2 tablespoons minced shallot

4 quarter-size slices peeled fresh ginger

2 cloves peeled garlic

4 medium (about 1 pound) peeled, halved, seeded, coarsely chopped tomatoes (see Note, page 195)

1¼ cups fat-free chicken or vegetable broth

½ cup unflavored soymilk

Salt and pepper to taste

Garnish:

¼ cup fresh basil leaves, cut in chiffonade (see Note below)

Heat olive oil in a 2-quart saucepan over medium heat. Add shallot and ginger and sauté until softened, about 1 minute.

Add garlic and tomatoes to the saucepan. Simmer until mixture begins to thicken, about 4 minutes. Remove slices of ginger. Add chicken broth and bring to a boil.

Carefully transfer soup to the bowl of a food processor or a blender jar. Process until smooth. Return to the saucepan. Add soymilk and simmer just until heated. Do not boil or soymilk will curdle. Season with salt and pepper and garnish with basil.

NOTE: The chiffonade cut is done by rolling the leaves lengthwise and slicing crosswise into thin slivers.

Tomato Factoid: California is the world's largest tomato producer, accounting for nearly half the world's processed tomato production.

Nutrient Analysis: per 1-cup serving

CALORIES: 82 PROTEIN: 4 grams CARBS.: 8 grams TOTAL FAT: 4 grams SAT. FAT: 1 gram
POLY. FAT: 1 gram MONO. FAT: 2 grams CHOLES.: 0 mg FIBER: 2 grams SODIUM: 59 mgs

Smoky Tomato Stew with Country Bread and Cannellini Beans

The addition of cannellini beans makes this version of Tuscan bread soup more substantial. Serve it warm or cold. A hint of chipotle chiles gives it a rich smoky flavor.

YIELD: 1½ QUARTS; 6 (1-CUP) SERVINGS
PREPARATION TIME: 35 MINUTES

1 tablespoon olive oil
¾ cup chopped red onion
1 teaspoon chopped chipotle chiles (see Note, page 63)
2 large minced garlic cloves
3½ cups fat-free chicken or vegetable broth
1 pound plum tomatoes, cored and coarsely chopped (about 5 plum tomatoes)
3 (¾-inch-thick) slices cubed whole-grain bread
1½ cups cooked cannellini beans or 1 (15-ounce) can, drained and rinsed
Salt and pepper to taste

Garnish:
⅓ cup slivered fresh basil, without stems
⅓ cup grated Parmesan cheese

Heat oil in a 3-quart saucepan over medium heat. Add onion and sauté 3 minutes. Add chiles, garlic, broth, tomatoes, and bread and bring soup to a boil. Reduce heat to medium low, cover, and simmer until bread is falling apart, about 5 minutes.

Transfer soup to the bowl of a food processor or a blender jar. Using on/off turns, blend to a coarse purée. Return mixture to saucepan. Add cannellini beans and bring to a simmer over low heat. Season with salt and pepper.

Distribute basil among six soup bowls. Ladle soup into bowls. Sprinkle with cheese.

NOTE: Chipotle chiles, canned in a spicy sauce called *adobo,* are available at Latin American markets, specialty foods stores, and some supermarkets. Leftover canned chiles can be transferred to a glass jar and stored in the refrigerator for up to 2 weeks. Dried chipotle chiles can be rehydrated and used instead of the canned ones.

Tomato Factoid: Studies have shown that cooked tomatoes have a higher concentration of lycopene than do raw tomatoes. When combined with a small amount of fat, the amount of lycopene the body absorbs is increased.

Nutrient Analysis: per 1-cup serving

CALORIES: 166   PROTEIN: 11 grams   CARBS.: 24 grams   TOTAL FAT: 2 grams   SAT. FAT: 1 gram
POLY. FAT: 0 gram   MONO. FAT: 1 gram   CHOLES.: 5 mgs   FIBER: 2 grams   SODIUM: 290 mgs

Roasted Tomato Curry with Gingered Garbanzo Beans and Baby Spinach

This Thai-inspired curry is loaded with fiber. Roasting the tomatoes and onions adds rich depth to the flavor. A great side dish, it holds its own as a complete meal when served with steamed whole grains or brown rice and a crisp green salad.

YIELD: 1½ QUARTS; 6 (1-CUP) SERVINGS
PREPARATION TIME: 1 HOUR

1½ pounds cored, peeled plum tomatoes, cut into 4 wedges each
1 large yellow onion, halved through root end, each half cut into
*   thin wedges*
Salt and pepper to taste
2 tablespoons olive oil
1 tablespoon peeled, minced fresh ginger

3 minced garlic cloves
1 tablespoon curry powder
¾ teaspoon ground coriander
¾ teaspoon ground cumin
1½ cups light coconut milk (see Notes below)
1 tablespoon fish sauce (see Notes below)
1 cup fat-free chicken or vegetable broth
1½ cups cooked garbanzo beans (chickpeas) or 1 (15-ounce) can,
    drained and rinsed
¾ cup (about 4 ounces) finely chopped fresh or frozen spinach
¼ cup chopped fresh cilantro, without stems

Roast tomatoes and onion: Preheat oven to 400 degrees Fahrenheit. Lightly coat a 15 x 10-inch baking sheet with olive oil spray. Combine tomato and onion wedges in a medium mixing bowl. Sprinkle with salt and pepper and drizzle with 1 tablespoon of the olive oil; toss to coat. Spread tomatoes and onion wedges in an even layer on prepared baking sheet. Roast until onion begins to brown, stirring occasionally, about 30 minutes. Set aside.

Heat remaining 1 tablespoon of oil in a 3-quart saucepan over medium heat. Add ginger and garlic and sauté, stirring, until light golden. Add curry powder, coriander, and cumin. Stir well and sauté until fragrant, 1 minute. Add coconut milk, tomato-onion mixture, and fish sauce and bring just to a boil. Remove from heat and carefully transfer to the bowl of a food processor or a blender jar. Process until smooth.

Return mixture to saucepan. Add broth, garbanzo beans, and spinach and heat until warmed. Season with salt and pepper. Sprinkle with cilantro.

NOTES: Light or "lite" coconut milk has less fat, fewer calories, and lighter flavor than regular coconut milk.

Fish sauce, also called *nuoc nam,* is available in Asian markets, specialty foods stores, and some supermarkets.

Tomato Factoid: If you're out of tomato sauce, you can convert a 3-ounce can of tomato paste into sauce by adding 1 cup water.

Nutrient Analysis: per 1-cup serving

CALORIES: 173   PROTEIN: 7 grams   CARBS.: 20 grams   TOTAL FAT: 8 grams   SAT. FAT: 2 grams
POLY. FAT: 1 gram   MONO. FAT: 3 grams   CHOLES.: 0 mg   FIBER: 5 grams   SODIUM: 293 mgs

Savory Moussaka with Pumate Béchamel

This classic meat and eggplant dish is loaded with lycopene. Ground turkey is simmered in richly seasoned tomatoes, and chunks of sun-dried tomatoes (known as *pumate* in Italian) pepper the creamy blanket of béchamel sauce. Allowing the flavors to meld intensifies the flavor. This moussaka is even more delicious the day after it's been baked, and it freezes well up to 1 month.

YIELD: 8 SERVINGS
PREPARATION TIME: 1 HOUR

Meat Mixture:
2 teaspoons olive oil
1 pound lean ground turkey or ground soy protein
1 cup chopped red onion
¾ cup dry red wine
1¾ cups (15 ounces) tomato sauce
1 tablespoon chopped fresh oregano or 1 teaspoon dried
1 teaspoon ground nutmeg
1 teaspoon ground cinnamon
1 tablespoon sorghum syrup or dark honey

Béchamel Sauce:
3 tablespoons olive oil
¼ cup unbleached all-purpose flour
¼ teaspoon ground pepper
2 minced garlic cloves

1½ cups unflavored soymilk
¾ cup fat-free chicken or vegetable broth
½ cup chopped green onion (green and white parts)
¾ cup finely chopped sun-dried tomatoes (pumate)
Salt and pepper to taste

1 medium eggplant (about 1¼ pounds), washed, halved lengthwise,
   and sliced crosswise into ¼-inch-thick rounds
Salt and pepper to taste
⅓ cup grated Parmesan cheese

Prepare meat mixture: Heat olive oil in large heavy saucepan over medium-high heat. Add turkey and onion. Cook, stirring to break up turkey, until it is no longer pink, about 5 minutes. Add wine, tomato sauce, oregano, spices, and sorghum syrup. Simmer, stirring occasionally, until mixture thickens and is almost dry, about 30 minutes. (Can be prepared 1 day ahead. Cover tightly and refrigerate.)

Preheat oven to 350 degrees Fahrenheit. Lightly coat a 13 x 9-inch glass baking dish with olive oil spray.

Prepare béchamel sauce: Heat olive oil in a 2-quart saucepan over medium heat. Whisk in flour and pepper. Cook 1 to 2 minutes, stirring constantly with a whisk. Add garlic and cook until softened; do not brown. Pour in soymilk and broth all at once. Simmer over low heat, stirring constantly, until thickened and bubbly. Remove from heat; stir in green onion and tomatoes. Season with salt and pepper. Set aside.

Assemble moussaka: Arrange half of eggplant in bottom of prepared dish. Season with salt and pepper. Add meat mixture and spread in an even layer. Top with remaining eggplant. Press down lightly with palm of your hand to evenly distribute. Season with salt and pepper. Pour hot béchamel sauce over the eggplant. Sprinkle with cheese.

Bake about 1 hour, or until golden and bubbling on edges. Cool 10 minutes before serving.

Tomato Factoid: It takes 17 pounds of fresh tomatoes to make 1 pound of dried tomatoes.

Nutrient Analysis: per 4½ x 3¼-inch piece

CALORIES: 274   PROTEIN: 16 grams   CARBS.: 19 grams   TOTAL FAT: 13 grams   SAT. FAT:

3 grams   POLY. FAT: 2 grams   MONO. FAT: 7 grams   CHOLES.: 48 mgs   FIBER: 5 grams

(Sol. 1 gram)   SODIUM: 461 mgs

Tomato Jam with Lemon and Basil

This unusual jam is a delicious way to celebrate the bounty of your harvest. Mound it on grilled bruschetta for a quick appetizer. I love to serve it as a condiment with cold poached salmon.

YIELD: 1½ CUPS; 12 (2-TABLESPOON) SERVINGS

PREPARATION TIME: 1 HOUR

> 2½ pounds (10 plum or about 5 large) peeled, seeded, coarsely chopped
>   ripe tomatoes
> 1 tablespoon grated lemon peel
> 3 tablespoons fresh lemon juice
> ½ teaspoon salt
> 1 cup sorghum syrup
> 2 tablespoons chopped fresh basil, without stems

Place in a 4-quart nonreactive saucepan. Add lemon peel, juice, and salt to tomatoes. Bring tomato mixture to a boil over medium heat. Reduce heat to low and simmer, stirring occasionally, until tomatoes have released most of their liquid but haven't lost their shape, about 12 minutes.

Slowly pour in sorghum syrup. Bring jam to a boil, stirring frequently, and boil until jam thickens, about 15 minutes. A candy thermometer should read 230 degrees Fahrenheit. You may also test by placing a drop of boiling liquid from the pan on to a cool plate. Allow to cool. If jam is ready, it will gel or thicken.

Remove from heat. Stir in the chopped basil. Pour into clean, sterilized jars and seal. Cool and refrigerate for up to 1 month.

Tomato Factoid: Grape tomatoes are the same size as cherry tomatoes and have nearly twice the sugar of a regular, big tomato.

Nutrient Analysis: per 2-tablespoon serving

CALORIES: 104 PROTEIN: 1 gram CARBS.: 25 grams TOTAL FAT: 0 gram SAT. FAT: 0 gram POLY. FAT: 0 gram MONO. FAT: 0 gram CHOLES.: 0 mg FIBER: 1 gram SODIUM: 108 mgs

Southwestern Barbecue Sauce with Chipotle Chiles

This tangy sauce is truly versatile. The perfect standby for a last-minute meal, it is an excellent marinade for grilled chicken or tofu. As a base for baked beans, it is incomparable. The recipe can be doubled, but the cooking time will be slightly longer. Chipotle, or smoked jalapeño, chiles impart a rich smoky flavor to the sauce. If unavailable, fresh jalapeño chiles can be used.

YIELD: 1 QUART; 16 (2-TABLESPOON) SERVINGS
PREPARATION TIME: 30 MINUTES

2 tablespoons olive oil
½ cup finely chopped red onion
1 minced garlic clove
2¾ cups (23 ounces) tomato sauce
½ cup fresh lemon juice
½ cup balsamic vinegar
½ cup sorghum syrup
2 tablespoons chili powder
1 tablespoon chopped chipotle chiles (see Note, page 63)

Heat oil in a 2-quart saucepan over medium heat. Add onion and sauté, stirring occasionally, until soft and translucent, about 3 minutes. Stir in garlic and sauté until softened; do not brown. Add remaining ingredients and simmer 20 minutes.

Tomato Factoid: Though *heirloom* is often perceived as a trendy moniker, it originally described a tomato variety that was nurtured (sometimes for generations) for prized characteristics, such as flavor.

Nutrient Analysis: per 2-tablespoon serving

CALORIES: 37 PROTEIN: 0 gram CARBS.: 7 grams TOTAL FAT: 1 gram SAT. FAT: 0 gram
POLY. FAT: 0 gram MONO. FAT: 1 gram CHOLES.: 0 mg FIBER: 1 gram SODIUM: 11 mgs

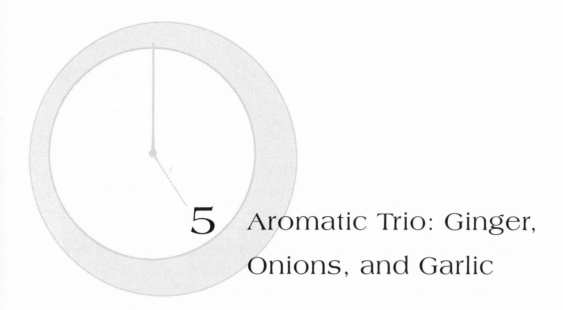

5 Aromatic Trio: Ginger, Onions, and Garlic

The pungent aroma of ginger, onions, and garlic, from a simmering pot of soup says something good is cooking. In a split second, one whiff conjures up the memory of a flavor, a moment, or a meal. The full-bodied richness of the fragrance reminds us that a splash of broth, a plump piece of fish, or a few crisp-tender vegetables are all we need for a quick and satisfying meal. On or off the fire, this dynamic trio doesn't simmer—it sizzles.

GINGER

It seamlessly crosses continents in lacquered sauces, robust chutneys, spicy stir-fries, exotic vinaigrettes, or pungent, frosty ice cream. The part of ginger that is used is the rhizome, or underground stem, a knobby, gnarly root that is peeled and minced before cooking. Sautéed, simmered, infused, baked, or fried, it has almost limitless applications. But beyond its incredible culinary diversity, it has medicinal properties that we rarely extol.

For centuries, Asian cultures have recognized ginger's curative wonders. From its fragrant scent in a steaming bowl of breakfast noodles to its peppery heat in a glass of bedtime tea, ginger is comforting at any hour. But as our internal clocks advance, mealtimes can be less pleasant. Age sometimes gives rise to disagreeable symptoms such as indigestion, gas, and even nausea. Make way; clear a prominent place for ginger in your kitchen. Its soothing, muscle-relaxing effects offer welcome respite to digestive woes. This is due to an antioxidant called *gingerol*. It also stimulates bile production from the gall bladder, thus enhancing digestion.

But that's not all. Two other phytochemicals, shogaol and zingerone, have antitussive and anti-inflammatory properties. This means they relieve cough and congestion from a cold or the flu. They are also known to minimize discomfort from the ravages of arthritis.

Ginger provides support to our internal line of antioxidant defense enzymes: superoxide dismutase, catalase, and glutathione peroxidase. This is thought to slow the oxidation of LDL cholesterol, promoting cardiovascular health and overall oxidative balance.

Heal thyself and expand your culinary repertoire with Amber Ginger Ale, Curried Chicken Stew, Spicy Ginger-Berry Biscotti, and Preserved Ginger.

ONIONS

The ancient Egyptians believed that the concentric rings of the onion symbolized eternal life. Who knew that modern science would prove their belief so prophetic?

The onion belongs to the Allium family, which also includes scallions, leeks, shallots, and garlic. There are few cultures throughout the world that don't regularly season their meals with a hint of one or a gargantuan dose of another. Thinly sliced chives on a steaming bowl of broth, a glistening mound of caramelized shallots, or a translucent onion that melts into the essence of a sauce; there are hundreds of ways to savor the flavors of the Allium family.

Where there's flavor, there's antiaging redemption. Quercetin, a phytochemical found in many green vegetables, is also prevalent in red and violet onions. Quercetin has several heart-healthy properties. Along with diallyl sulfide, it fights cancer. Both are antioxidants, and both promote overall oxidative balance. Sulfonate compounds are prominent in onions, chives, leeks, and shallots and are similar to the sulfur compounds found in cabbage and cruciferous vegetables. They interact beneficially with our liver's detoxification processes, promoting aggressive attack on cancer-causing substances.

Slow your clock and savor the flavors of Scalloped Tomatoes with Caramelized Onions or Chicken Shwarma in Warm Pitas with Tomato-Cucumber Salad.

GARLIC

Folklore has exalted garlic for centuries for its ability to ward off disease *and* evil spirits. Ancient civilizations culled their prescriptive stash from the garden, not a medicine chest. Garlic was a curative for a slew of symptoms ranging from fatigue to asthma. These customs didn't die. Researchers continue to stir up clues substantiating garlic's preventive and therapeutic vigor. This savory bulb contains hundreds of compounds that defend cells against attack by age-promoting free radicals.

Many of garlic's beneficial properties relate to heart health. Studies reflect that garlic's saponin component often lowers triglycerides and cholesterol by as much as 10 percent. This may be the result of both decreased absorption and decreased production of cholesterol by the liver. This phytochemical also decreases platelet aggregation, or blood clotting, thus decreasing risk for stroke. In addition, there are indications that it may contribute to lower blood pressure.

Other studies reveal that the diverse range of phytochemicals contained in garlic has powerful antioxidant benefits that not only contribute to oxidative balance but also have antibacterial, antiviral, and antifungal properties. We don't understand the mechanisms of all of garlic's healing powers, but they appear to enhance our immune system in ways that fight cancer cells. They also stimulate immune responses by activating cells that specifically target tumor cells.

Taste a remedy from a recipe with *Baba Ghanouj* (Roasted Eggplant Purée), Creamy Onion Soup with Roasted Garlic, and Thyme and Roasted Garlic Purée.

Baba Ghanouj (Roasted Eggplant Purée)

The flavor is regal and the texture of this creamy appetizer is truly imperial. It's no wonder, since my inspiration for the recipe came from Chef Sahd, who cooks for the Saudi royal family. His addictive Middle Eastern eggplant dip is traditionally served with warm pita bread and an assortment of salads. It's a great make-ahead hors d'oeuvre. It keeps refrigerated for several days.

YIELD: 4 CUPS; 32 (2-TABLESPOON) SERVINGS
PREPARATION TIME: 1 HOUR

2 large eggplants (about 1½ pounds each)
⅓ cup fresh lemon juice
½ cup tahini (see Note, page 46)
1 tablespoon ground cumin
1 tablespoon minced garlic
2 teaspoons white wine vinegar
1 cup fat-free plain yogurt or plain soy yogurt (see Note, page 75)
2 teaspoons salt (optional)

Garnish:
¼ cup finely chopped Italian parsley, without stems

Wash and dry the eggplant. Cut off stem end. Pierce skin with a fork to prevent eggplant from bursting during roasting.

For stovetop roasting or grilling: Place eggplant directly on grill rack or over gas burner at medium heat. Grill for about 18 minutes, turning frequently to cook evenly. Remove from heat when eggplant has become very soft. Set aside roasted eggplant to cool.

For oven roasting: Position rack in middle of oven and preheat oven to 350 degrees Fahrenheit. Lightly coat a 15 x 10-inch baking sheet with olive oil spray. Place eggplant on prepared baking sheet and bake for about 40 minutes, turning eggplant three or four times to roast evenly. Remove from oven when eggplant becomes soft.

Assemble dish: When cool enough to handle, peel eggplant and discard skin. Remove most of the seeds and cut eggplant into chunks.

Combine remaining ingredients except parsley, eggplant, and salt, in a blender jar or the bowl of a food processor. Purée until smooth. If mixture is too thick, add hot water by tablespoons to achieve the right consistency. Add eggplant chunks and process just until smooth.

Adjust seasoning with salt if necessary. Garnish with finely chopped parsley.

NOTE: Soy yogurt is available in most grocery stores and health food stores. Using soy yogurt may result in a slightly sweeter taste.

Sesame Factoid: Sesame seeds are an excellent source of protein and calcium.

Nutrient Analysis: per 2-tablespoon serving

CALORIES: 32   PROTEIN: 2 grams   CARBS.: 3 grams   TOTAL FAT: 3 grams   SAT. FAT: 0 gram

POLY. FAT: 1 gram   MONO. FAT: 1 gram   CHOLES.: 0 mg   FIBER: 1 gram   SODIUM: 173 mgs

Creamy Onion Soup with Roasted Garlic and Thyme

This rustic soup is so robust and creamy, it could also be used as a sauce with chicken or fish. Serve with crusty whole-grain bread for a hearty meal on a cold winter night.

YIELD: 7 CUPS; 6 (1¼-CUP) SERVINGS

PREPARATION TIME: 45 MINUTES

1 tablespoon olive oil

⅓ cup peeled whole garlic cloves (1 large head)

4 medium (1½ pounds) thinly sliced yellow onions

1½ teaspoons chopped fresh oregano or ½ teaspoon dried

2 tablespoons balsamic vinegar

3 cups fat-free chicken or vegetable broth

½ cup unflavored soymilk

Salt and pepper to taste

Chopped chives

Heat oil in a heavy 4-quart saucepan over medium-low heat. Add garlic and cook, stirring frequently, until light golden brown and caramelized, about 6 minutes. Do not brown garlic beyond this, or it will be bitter. Add onions and cook, stirring frequently, until onions are softened and just starting to brown, about 10 minutes. Add oregano and balsamic vinegar and sauté 2 minutes longer. Add broth and bring to a boil. Reduce heat and simmer, uncovered, 5 minutes.

Transfer soup to the bowl of a food processor or to a blender jar and process soup until very smooth and creamy. Stir in soymilk. Return soup to pan and heat thoroughly but do not boil.

Season with salt and pepper. Ladle into bowls and sprinkle with chives.

> *Oregano Factoid:* A phytochemical in oregano called *carvacrol* has exhibited antibacterial properties. Oregano, with its antioxidant powers, is renowned in the Mediterranean region for its ability to preserve foods.

Nutrient Analysis: per 1¼-cup serving

CALORIES: 100   PROTEIN: 5 grams   CARBS.: 13 grams   TOTAL FAT: 3 grams   SAT. FAT: 0 gram
POLY. FAT: 1 gram   MONO. FAT: 2 grams   CHOLES.: 0 mg   FIBER: 2 grams (Sol. 1 gram)
SODIUM: 93 mgs

Curried Chicken Stew

A fragrant blend of spices punctuates this robust stew. Serve it hot over steaming brown rice or whole grains for a hearty meal. Add an additional cup of broth and serve it as a soup. For a vegetarian version, replace the chicken with garbanzo beans or cubes of firm tofu.

YIELD: 2 QUARTS; 8 (1-CUP) SERVINGS
PREPARATION TIME: 40 MINUTES

1 tablespoon olive oil
2 cups finely chopped red onion

2 tablespoons peeled, finely chopped fresh ginger

2 cloves minced garlic

1 cup peeled, halved, seeded, chopped tomatoes (see Note, page 195)

1 tablespoon ground coriander

1 tablespoon ground cumin

½ teaspoon ground cardamom

¼ teaspoon ground cinnamon

3 cups fat-free low-sodium chicken or vegetable broth

1 (12-ounce) sweet potato, peeled and cut into ½-inch dice
   (about 2 cups)

1 pound boneless, skinless chicken breasts, cut into ½-inch cubes

Salt and pepper to taste

¼ cup chopped fresh cilantro, without stems

Heat oil in a large heavy pot over medium heat. Add onions and cook, stirring occasionally, until onions are tender but not brown, about 10 minutes.

Add ginger and garlic; sauté until fragrant, about 1 minute. Do not brown garlic. Add tomatoes and simmer 5 minutes. Add spices and cook until very fragrant, about 1 minute.

Add chicken broth and bring to a boil. Stir in sweet potato and simmer for about 4 minutes.

Add chicken and simmer until cooked through, about 5 minutes. Season with salt and pepper.

Serve hot, sprinkled with cilantro.

Onion Factoid: Eye tearing caused by cutting onions can be prevented by chilling them beforehand. The cold inactivates the offending compound (*propanethial-s-oxide*) and prevents it from becoming airborne.

Nutrient Analysis: per 1-cup serving

CALORIES: 159   PROTEIN: 17 grams   CARBS.: 16 grams   TOTAL FAT: 3 grams   SAT. FAT: 0 gram

POLY. FAT: 0 gram   MONO. FAT: 2 grams   CHOLES.: 33 mgs   FIBER: 3 grams   SODIUM: 109 mgs

Chicken Shwarma in Warm Pitas with Tomato-Cucumber Salad

This rendition of a classic Middle Eastern sandwich is simply sublime. Tender shreds of perfectly seasoned chicken are wrapped in warm pita bread and covered with a crisp salad of tomato and cucumber. Lemon Tahini Sauce (page 46) is the ultimate condiment to drizzle on this heavenly sandwich.

Yield: 8 sandwiches

Preparation time: 1 hour plus marinating overnight

Marinade:
1 medium yellow onion, cut into eighths
¼ cup fresh lemon or lime juice
2 tablespoons white vinegar
2 tablespoons extra-virgin olive oil
2 tablespoons tahini (see Note, page 46)
2 tablespoons peeled, coarsely chopped fresh ginger
3 peeled garlic cloves
1 teaspoon ground cumin
½ teaspoon ground ginger
½ teaspoon ground cardamom
¼ teaspoon ground cloves
¼ teaspoon ground cinnamon
¼ teaspoon ground nutmeg
¼ teaspoon ground pepper

2 pounds boneless, skinless chicken breasts, cut into ½-inch-wide strips

Tomato-Cucumber Salad:

½ cup finely chopped cilantro, without stems
½ cup finely chopped fresh mint, without stems
3 medium seeded and diced tomatoes
1 peeled, seeded, diced English cucumber
1 seeded and diced yellow bell pepper
Salt and pepper to taste

8 pieces (6-inch-diameter) whole-wheat pita bread, halved
½ head thinly sliced romaine lettuce (about 3 cups)

Prepare marinade: Combine all marinade ingredients in a blender or food processor and puree. Mixture will be a thick paste. Pour marinade into a 3-quart nonreactive mixing bowl. Add chicken and stir to coat with marinade. Cover and marinate in the refrigerator for 12 hours or overnight.

Prepare salad: Combine salad ingredients in a bowl, season to taste, and set aside.

Wrap pita bread in aluminum foil and place in preheated 250-degree Fahrenheit oven for about 20 minutes or until warmed.

Blot excess marinade from the chicken to prevent burning. Lightly coat a nonstick sauté pan with olive oil cooking spray. Cook chicken in batches over medium-high heat until cooked through, about 4 minutes. Keep cooked chicken warm in a covered container. (Chicken may also be placed on skewers and cooked on grill.)

Place some of the lettuce inside each pita bread, add 2 or 3 strips of chicken, and top with salad.

Onion Factoid: The tearjerker in onions is a compound called *propanethial-s-oxide,* which is released in a vapor when onions are cut. When the vapor comes in contact with the eye, it is converted to a form of sulfuric acid, which produces the stinging sensation and subsequent tears.

Nutrient Analysis: per sandwich

Calories: 195   Protein: 17 grams   Carbs.: 23 grams   Total fat: 4 grams   Sat. fat: 1 gram
Poly. fat: 1 gram   Mono. fat: 2 grams   Choles.: 33 mgs   Fiber: 3 grams (Sol. 1 gram)
Sodium: 213 mgs

Scalloped Tomatoes with Caramelized Onions

Silky and sweet, caramelized onions add a rustic touch to unadorned tomatoes. Serve with roast chicken and a green vegetable. This is a great dish for a potluck, as it can be assembled a day ahead of time and baked just before serving.

YIELD: 1½ QUARTS; 8 (¾-CUP) SERVINGS
PREPARATION TIME: 1 HOUR

Caramelized Onions:
1 tablespoon olive oil
2 large onions, halved lengthwise and cut crosswise into ⅛-inch-thick
*   slices*
¼ teaspoon salt
⅛ teaspoon ground pepper
⅓ cup fat-free chicken or vegetable broth
2 tablespoons balsamic vinegar

Sauce:
¼ cup olive oil
¼ cup unbleached all-purpose flour
2 cups fat-free chicken or vegetable broth
1 teaspoon Italian seasoning (mixed dry herbs such as oregano, thyme,
*   and basil)*
Salt and pepper to taste

2 pounds plum tomatoes (10 to 12 tomatoes)
⅓ cup coarsely grated Parmigiana Reggiano cheese
⅓ cup fresh bread crumbs

Preheat oven to 375 degrees Fahrenheit. Lightly coat a 2-quart soufflé or baking dish with olive oil cooking spray.

Prepare onions: Heat oil in a large skillet over medium-high heat. Add onions, salt, and pepper; cook, stirring frequently, until onions begin to brown, about 12 minutes. Add broth and vinegar. Reduce heat to medium; simmer, stirring occasionally, until juices are nearly dry, about 12 minutes.

Meanwhile, prepare sauce: Heat olive oil in a heavy saucepan over medium-low heat and whisk in flour to make a paste. Cook the paste, whisking, about 2 minutes. Add broth in a stream, continuing to whisk. Bring sauce to a boil, reduce heat, and simmer until thickened, about 2 minutes. Remove pan from heat and stir in seasoning and salt and pepper. Set aside.

Core tomatoes and cut crosswise into about ¼-inch-thick slices. Combine cheese and bread crumbs in a small mixing bowl.

Assemble dish: In prepared baking dish, layer one-third of tomatoes, one-third of onions, and one-third of sauce. Repeat layers two more times. Sprinkle bread crumb mixture on top and bake, uncovered, for 35 minutes, or until top is golden. Serve warm.

Tomato Factoid: Refrigerating fresh tomatoes causes them to lose up to 30 percent of their flavor. Store them at room temperature for optimal taste and texture.

Nutrient Analysis: per ¾-cup serving

CALORIES: 186   PROTEIN: 6 grams   CARBS.: 18 grams   TOTAL FAT: 10 grams   SAT. FAT: 2 grams

POLY. FAT: 1 gram   MONO. FAT: 7 grams   CHOLES.: 3 mgs   FIBER: 2 grams (Sol. 1 gram)

SODIUM: 210 mgs

Roasted Garlic Purée

Roasted garlic is sophisticated in its simplicity. The richness of this luscious spread is complemented by crusty chunks of whole-grain bread. Roasted Garlic Purée can be spread on bread or crackers or stirred into soups, mashed potatoes, vinaigrettes, or sauces.

YIELD: 6 HEADS GARLIC; 6 SERVINGS
PREPARATION TIME: 1 HOUR

6 large heads garlic
2 tablespoons extra-virgin olive oil
Salt and pepper to taste
1 tablespoon fresh lemon juice (optional)

Preheat oven to 350 degrees Fahrenheit.

Cut off tips of the garlic heads, barely exposing the cloves. Remove outermost layer of skin from garlic heads but do not separate the cloves.

Place garlic heads in a shallow 8-inch-square baking dish, and drizzle with olive oil. Season with salt and pepper. Cover with aluminum foil and bake about 40 minutes or until very soft.

Let stand until cool enough to handle. Roasted garlic may be squeezed out of the skins and eaten as is. For a smoother texture, process garlic in a food processor with salt, pepper, and lemon juice (if using) for 30 seconds.

Garlic Factoid: A bulb (also called a *head*) of garlic typically consists of 12–16 cloves. One medium clove equals ½ teaspoon of minced garlic. Of all the vegetables, garlic contains the highest amount of the antioxidant selenium.

Nutrient Analysis: per roasted garlic head

CALORIES: 92   PROTEIN: 3 grams   CARBS.: 14 grams   TOTAL FAT: 4 grams   SAT. FAT: 0 gram

POLY. FAT: 0 gram   MONO. FAT: 3 grams   CHOLES.: 0 mg   FIBER: 1 gram   SODIUM: 7 mgs

Preserved Ginger

Unlike crystallized or candied ginger, which is firm and dry, preserved ginger is cooked and then stored in a sweet syrup. In this case, sorghum syrup is used instead of sugar. The dark, intensely flavored syrup is retained and stored with the ginger rather than drying the slices separately. It adds sparkle to a bowl of hot cereal and can be used in most recipes requiring crystallized ginger. I am not sure how long it keeps; in my house it never lasts long enough to find out.

YIELD: ¾ CUP

PREPARATION TIME: 1 HOUR 15 MINUTES

> *1 cup (¼-inch-thick) slices peeled fresh ginger*
> *1 cup water*
> *½ cup sorghum syrup*

Bring 2 cups water to boil in a 1-quart saucepan. Add ginger slices, reduce heat, and simmer for 5 minutes. Drain. Repeat boiling and draining.

Add 1 cup water and sorghum syrup to the saucepan and bring to a boil. Add drained ginger, reduce heat, and simmer until syrup is thick and dark, about 1 hour. Watch carefully and stir occasionally so that the syrup doesn't burn.

Transfer ginger and syrup to a small clean jar. Keep refrigerated.

Ginger Factoid: Fresh ginger can be used in cooking in a variety of forms: sliced, shredded, minced, grated, juiced, pounded, and even unpeeled. It is also dried and ground into a spice.

Nutrient Analysis: per tablespoon

CALORIES: 48　PROTEIN: 0 gram　CARBS.: 11 grams　TOTAL FAT: 0 gram　SAT. FAT: 0 gram
POLY. FAT: 0 gram　MONO. FAT: 0 gram　CHOLES.: 0 mg　FIBER: 0 gram　SODIUM: 2 mgs

Spicy Ginger-Berry Biscotti

These biscotti are a bit more delicate than some of their Italian counterparts. Slivers of dried plums or dried cranberries substitute nicely for the blueberries.

YIELD: ABOUT 36 BISCOTTI
PREPARATION TIME: 1 HOUR

½ cup sorghum syrup
⅓ cup olive oil
1 teaspoon grated lemon or orange peel
1 tablespoon pure vanilla extract
1 large egg
1¾ cups unbleached all-purpose flour
½ cup sorghum flour
2 tablespoons stone-ground cornmeal
1 teaspoon baking powder
1 teaspoon ground ginger
¼ teaspoon salt
¼ cup finely chopped crystallized ginger (see Note, page 119)
⅓ cup finely chopped dried blueberries
½ cup chopped, toasted walnuts (see Note, page 31)

Preheat oven to 350 degrees Fahrenheit. Lightly coat a 15 x 10-inch baking sheet with olive oil spray.

Whisk together sorghum syrup, olive oil, lemon peel, vanilla, and egg in a medium mixing bowl. Combine the flours, cornmeal, baking powder, ground ginger, and salt in a large mixing bowl. Make a well in the center and pour in the liquid ingredients. Stir just to combine. Stir in chopped ginger, blueberries, and walnuts. Dough will be soft.

Transfer dough to a lightly floured work surface. Form into 2 rolls about 10 inches long and 1½ inches in diameter. Press rolls with palm of your hand to flatten to a 1-inch thickness. Place biscotti rolls on prepared baking sheet and bake 20 minutes. Transfer to a wire rack to cool for 10 minutes.

While biscotti rolls are still warm, slice each of them diagonally with a serrated knife into about 18 (½-inch-thick) slices (for a total of about 36 slices).

Place biscotti, cut side down, on an ungreased 15 x 10-inch baking sheet and return to oven to bake for 20 minutes. Remove from baking sheet; cool completely on wire racks.

Ginger Factoid: Though often simply referred to as a "root," ginger is better described as a *rhizome,* which is a tuberlike stem that grows underground with roots of its own.

Nutrient Analysis: per biscotti

Calories: 66   Protein: 10 grams   Carbs.: 10 grams   Total fat: 2 grams   Sat. fat: 0 gram

Poly. fat: 0 gram   Mono. fat: 2 grams   Choles.: 5 mgs   Fiber: 1 gram   Sodium: 49 mgs

Amber Ginger Ale

This pungent extract is a great way to get an antioxidant fix between meals. For a supercharged sipper, replace the sparkling water with a vibrantly hued fruit juice or green iced tea.

Yield: 1½ pints syrup; 7 (10-ounce) servings

Preparation time: 15 minutes

Ginger Syrup:
3 cups water
½ cup peeled, grated fresh ginger

2 tablespoons fresh lemon juice
2 tablespoons pure vanilla extract
½ cup sorghum syrup

Ginger Ale:
Ginger Syrup (above)
2 quarts chilled sparkling or carbonated water
Ice cubes

Prepare syrup: Bring ginger and water to a rapid boil in a 2-quart saucepan over medium-high heat. Boil 10 minutes. Remove from heat, strain ginger through a fine sieve, and pour liquid into a 1-quart jar. Stir in lemon juice, vanilla, and sorghum syrup; let cool. Store syrup in refrigerator for up to 2 weeks.

Prepare ginger ale: Add syrup to sparkling water. Add ice and stir. For 1 serving, add ¼ cup of syrup to 8 ounces sparkling or carbonated water.

> *Ginger Factoid:* Ginger is a member of the Zingiberaceae family of plants, which also includes the spice turmeric. Only one species of ginger, called *Zingiber officinale* (official ginger), is actually used for culinary purposes.

Nutrient Analysis: per 10-ounce serving

CALORIES: 83   PROTEIN: 0 gram   CARBS.: 18 grams   TOTAL FAT: 0 gram   SAT. FAT: 0 gram
POLY. FAT: 0 gram   MONO. FAT: 0 gram   CHOLES.: 0 mg   FIBER: 0 gram   SODIUM: 2 mgs

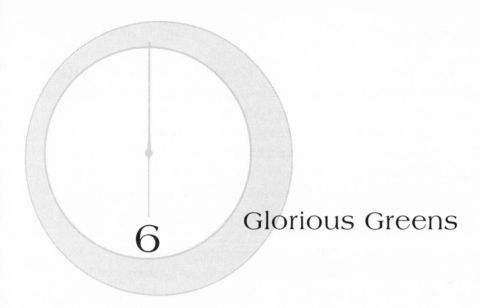

6 Glorious Greens

Their common color is a brilliant disguise for the magnificent array of textures and tastes that this powerful vegetable family embraces. Peppery, earthy, buttery, pungent—their flavors are as diverse as they are satisfying. It's no surprise that their antiaging properties offer a broad spectrum of benefits.

AVOCADOS

The voluptuous avocado embodies the sensual side of food. For centuries, its buttery texture and rich, nutty flavor have seduced palates and civilizations alike. The ancient Aztecs' love affair with avocados transcended mere sustenance; it was a passion deeply rooted in the faith of its aphrodisiac prowess.

Our infatuation is more modern. In the '70s, the nomadic avocado stormed the American party scene in the guise of a trendy dip. *Guacamole* was transformed from an unfamiliar Spanish name to a household word. For many of us, the creamy appetizer was the *only* way to enjoy this celebrated fruit. But just as our addiction kicked in, the next decade ushered in the news that fat-laden diets promote heart disease. We longed to kill the messenger, because our favorite rich foods had to go. We bid adiós to the avocado.

It's time to rekindle your passion and let the sparks fly. The avocado has earned a preferential place on your table, and, once again, it has everything to do with antiaging. Avocados still derive 75 percent of their calories from fat, so we need to indulge with moderation, but most of their fat is monounsaturated, which means it lowers LDL, the *least desirable* cholesterol, and that's only the beginning.

Like our favorite chocolates, the dark exterior of a ripe avocado conceals the wonderful surprises of its creamy interior. Lutein, a pale-green pigment, is a phytochemical that acts as a filter to protect the eye from potentially damaging forms of light. Consequently, lutein appears to be associated with protection against *macular degeneration,* the leading cause of blindness in aging adults.

Phytosterols are another magic secret in avocados. Though found primarily in nuts and seeds, two phytosterols, beta-sitosterol and campesterol, are also found in avocados, and they are similar in structure to cholesterol. Their cholesterol-cloning property enables them to simulate cholesterol's presence in the body, thus decreasing the amount of cholesterol produced and absorbed, thereby promoting cardiovascular health. Don't be surprised if your next batch of guacamole tastes better.

"A quarter of an avocado has about 80 calories, so use it instead of mayonnaise to dress up a sandwich or spread it on a whole-grain bagel instead of cream cheese," suggests Susan Bowerman, M.S., R.D., assistant director of the UCLA Center for Human Nutrition. You can also taste its antiaging richness in Sassy Tomato-Avocado Soup.

SPINACH

A few notches across the color spectrum are other shades of green with equally amazing benefits. Spinach boasts the highest quercetin levels of any vegetable or fruit. Quercetin is a powerful antioxidant and a flavonoid. In addition to fighting cancer-promoting invaders, quercetin also interferes with the oxidation of LDL cholesterol (which promotes artery blockage), thus promoting cardiovascular health.

Spinach has also shown remarkable promise in reversing nerve and behavioral deficits related to aging of the brain. Among a variety of high-antioxidant fruits and vegetables, spinach was the most potent in protecting certain types of nerve cells in the brain against the effects of aging. Stash away some stamina and taste the new flavors of an old favorite in *Saag Paneer* (Creamy Spinach with Peppery Cheese).

CRUCIFEROUS VEGETABLES

Broccoli belongs to the cruciferous vegetable family, which also includes cabbage, sprouts, and kale. But broccoli is the patriarch of this family in terms of its diversity of antiaging ammo, including sulforaphane, beta-carotene, lutein, and quercetin, to name a few. But let's give some meaning to this phytochemical mumbo jumbo.

Sulfur compounds are distinctive to all cruciferous vegetables. They supply their characteristic pungent aroma. Cooking intensifies their odor *and* their protective powers. Once eaten, the sulfur compounds convert to one of several products in the body. Each of those products has different structures and, subsequently, distinguishing antiaging benefits. One group of sulfur compounds, called *indoles,* is thought to activate liver enzymes with detoxifying properties to assert their action over potential cancer-causing substances. Cabbage and broccoli are particularly rich in indoles. It is important to note that the light-hued crucifers, such as cauliflower, boast similar compounds but in different proportions.

Kale is another form of cabbage and an antiaging powerhouse. It promotes cardiovascular health as a rich source of potassium and calcium. Together, these nutrients promote a reduced risk of stroke by regulating blood pressure. Kale's robust flavors are easy to enjoy in a quick sauté or stir-fry.

Another group of sulfur compounds, the *isothiocyanates,* is found in mustard greens and seeds, daikon, horseradish, and wasabi. Like the indoles, these phytochemicals have similar cancer-fighting effects. Crispy Kale Croquettes, Curried Creamed Cabbage, Asian Chicken Salad, Broccoli-Dill Soup, Nutty Glazed Brussels Sprouts, and Southern-Style Mustard Greens are your tickets to taste the star voltage of cruciferous vegetables.

WATERCRESS

Watercress isn't prominent on most shopping lists, but that could change. This peppery leafy green is loaded with phenyl ethyl isothiocyanate (PEITC). PEITC has powerful anticancer effects, particularly in the case of lung cancer, by preventing activation of carcinogenic substances found in cigarette smoke and other air pollutants. The deep emerald pigments of watercress also contain rich reserves of an omega-3 fatty acid called *alpha-linolenic acid* (ALA), as well as lutein and xeaxanthin. Watercress is a great alternative to lettuce in a sandwich or a salad such as Watercress and Cranberry Salad with Roasted Onion Dressing.

LETTUCE

The lettuce family may not be as rich in phytochemicals as most of the green vegetables, but it is an excellent source of fiber and B vitamins. Romaine is the exception to the rule in terms of its antiaging profile. Romaine contains significant amounts of lutein and xeaxanthin, promoting the longevity of our vision. Recharge your clock with the robust flavors of Egyptian Eggplant Salad.

Sassy Tomato-Avocado Soup

This velvety soup is a unique fusion of flavors. It only takes minutes to make because it uses tomato juice, which has been cooked. Heating tomato juice not only extends the shelf life but also concentrates the lycopene. Serve in chilled bowls garnished with a fresh lime wedge.

YIELD: 1¼ QUARTS; 6 (1-CUP) SERVINGS
PREPARATION TIME: 10 MINUTES

4 cups tomato juice
2 tablespoons finely chopped celery
1 tablespoon finely chopped onion
3 tablespoons fresh lime juice
2 tablespoons Worcestershire sauce
2 tablespoons Dijon mustard
2 tablespoon tahini (see Note, page 46)
1½ ripe medium avocados
¼ cup fresh lime juice
Salt and pepper to taste

Garnish:

¼ cup chopped fresh cilantro, without stems

Combine tomato juice, celery, onion, lime juice, Worcestershire sauce, mustard, and tahini in a blender or food processor. Purée until smooth. Season with salt and pepper. Cover and refrigerate until chilled or up to a day in advance.

Before serving, peel and pit the avocados; cut into ½-inch cubes. Toss avocado cubes with the remaining lime juice. Divide the avocado among six serving bowls.

Pour cold tomato mixture over avocados, about ¾ cup of the tomato mixture per bowl. Serve chilled. Garnish with fresh cilantro.

Avocado Factoid: Compared ounce for ounce, avocados have one of the highest fiber contents of all fresh fruits.

Nutrient Analysis: per 1-cup serving

CALORIES: 152 PROTEIN: 4 grams CARBS.: 14 grams TOTAL FAT: 11 grams
SAT. FAT: 2 grams POLY. FAT: 2 grams MONO. FAT: 6 grams CHOLES.: 0 mg
FIBER: 4 grams (Sol. 1 gram) SODIUM: 169 mgs

Broccoli-Dill Soup with Lemon and Tahini

The rich flavors of this creamy soup disguise the fact that it's remarkably light.

YIELD: 1½ QUARTS; 6 (1-CUP) SERVINGS
PREPARATION TIME: 45 MINUTES

1 tablespoon olive oil
1½ cups chopped yellow onion
1 teaspoon mustard seeds

½ cup coarsely ground bulgur

4 cups fat-free chicken or vegetable broth

1 tablespoon chopped fresh dill or 1 teaspoon dried

2 cups bite-size broccoli pieces (about 8 ounces)

¼ cup pitted, chopped ripe olives

1 tablespoon tahini (see Note, page 46)

1 teaspoon grated fresh lemon peel or minced Preserved Lemon Peel
*   (see Notes, pages 47–48)*

Salt and pepper to taste

Heat olive oil in a 3-quart saucepan over medium heat. Add onions and sauté until onions are just beginning to brown, about 7 minutes.

Add mustard seeds and bulgur and sauté about 3 minutes, stirring frequently. Carefully add broth and bring mixture to a boil. Reduce heat to low and simmer 10 minutes.

Add dill and broccoli and cook until broccoli is just tender, about 4 minutes. Stir in olives, tahini, and lemon peel and season with salt and pepper. Serve immediately.

Broccoli Factoid: Broccoli contains a compound called *sulforaphane,* which has shown promising anticancer effects. Current studies are now focusing on broccoli sprouts due to their particularly high-antioxidant activity.

Nutrient Analysis: per 1-cup serving

CALORIES: 130　PROTEIN: 8 grams　CARBS.: 16 grams　TOTAL FAT: 5 grams　SAT. FAT: 1 gram

POLY. FAT: 1 gram　MONO. FAT: 3 grams　CHOLES.: 0 mg　FIBER: 4 grams (Sol. 0.8 gram)

SODIUM: 177 mgs

Watercress and Cranberry Salad with Roasted Onion Dressing

Peppery watercress is a welcome change from lettuce in this salad of many textures and flavors. Try it with different nuts and berries, too. Extra dressing keeps well in the refrigerator for up to 1 week.

YIELD: 8 SERVINGS

PREPARATION TIME: 50 MINUTES

Roasted Onion Dressing:
1 medium red onion (about 8 ounces)
¼ cup plus 1 teaspoon olive oil
¼ cup fresh lime juice
1 tablespoon Dijon mustard
3 tablespoons balsamic vinegar
Salt and pepper to taste

Watercress and Cranberry Salad:
1 medium red apple
1 teaspoon fresh lime juice
4 cups watercress, washed, trimmed, dried
1½ cups dried cranberries or blueberries
⅓ cup chopped, toasted walnuts (see Note, page 31)

Prepare dressing: Preheat oven to 400 degrees Fahrenheit. Peel onion and cut into eight wedges. Place onion, cut side down, on baking sheet. Drizzle with 1 teaspoon of the olive oil. Bake for 15 minutes. Turn onion over and bake until brown and caramelized, about 15 minutes longer. Set aside to cool.

Place onion in bowl of a food processor. Add lime juice, mustard, and vinegar. Process until smooth and thick. (Add 1 tablespoon water if mixture is too thick to process.) Add the remaining ¼ cup olive oil in a thin stream. Season with salt and pepper. Set aside. There will be about 1¼ cups of dressing.

Prepare salad: Cut apple in half lengthwise and remove core. Cut halves crosswise into ¼-inch-thick slices. Stack the slices and cut crosswise into ⅛-inch-wide slices, forming thin matchsticks. In a large mixing bowl, toss apple sticks in lime juice. Set aside.

Add watercress, cranberries, and nuts to the apple. Add enough dressing to coat greens, about 3 tablespoons; toss well.

Divide salad equally among eight plates. Serve immediately. Pass extra dressing separately.

Watercress Factoid: Watercress contains many antioxidants, including *rhamnetin,* a flavonol that has shown remarkable strength in fighting cancer tumor cells in research studies.

Nutrient Analysis: per serving

CALORIES: 122 PROTEIN: 2 grams CARBS.: 20 grams TOTAL FAT: 4 grams SAT. FAT: 0 gram
POLY. FAT: 2 grams MONO. FAT: 2 grams CHOLES.: 0 mg FIBER: 3 grams (Sol. 0.4 gram)
SODIUM: 16 mgs

Egyptian Eggplant Salad

The simple earthiness of this large salad melds the flavors of Eastern and Western seasonings. It takes only a few minutes to assemble, though the preparation of the ingredients takes longer. It's a great make-ahead dish for a barbecue or potluck.

YIELD: ABOUT 12 CUPS; 8 (1½-CUP) SERVINGS
PREPARATION TIME: 1 HOUR

Salad:
2 large eggplants (about 1½ pounds each)
1½ heads romaine lettuce

1 medium red bell pepper, cut into fine dice
½ medium green bell pepper, cut into fine dice
1 peeled, seeded English cucumber, cut into fine dice (2 cups)
1 cup chopped green onion (green and white parts)
½ cup chopped fresh Italian parsley, without stems
½ cup chopped fresh mint, without stems

Dressing:
2 tablespoons minced garlic
¼ cup fresh lemon juice
2 tablespoons ground cumin
1½ teaspoons salt (optional)
½ teaspoon red pepper flakes (optional)
½ cup extra-virgin olive oil
Salt and pepper to taste

Prepare salad: Wash and dry eggplants. Cut off stem ends. Pierce skin with a fork to prevent eggplants from bursting during roasting.

For stovetop roasting or grilling: Place eggplants directly on grill rack or over gas burner at medium heat. Grill for about 18 minutes, turning frequently to cook evenly. Remove from heat when eggplants have become very soft. Set aside roasted eggplants to cool.

For oven roasting: Position rack in middle of oven and preheat oven to 350 degrees Fahrenheit. Lightly coat a 15 x 10-inch baking sheet with olive oil spray. Place eggplants on prepared baking sheet and bake for about 40 minutes, turning eggplants three or four times to roast evenly. Remove from oven when eggplants have become soft. When cool enough to handle, peel the skin of the eggplants and discard. Remove most of the seeds and cut eggplants into chunks.

Prepare dressing: Mash garlic with lemon juice until smooth. Add cumin and salt and red pepper flakes (if using). Add oil in a thin stream, whisking until it is completely incorporated. There will be about ¾ cup of dressing.

Assemble salad: Wash and dry romaine. Cut or tear romaine into bite-size pieces and place in a large mixing bowl. Add remaining chopped vegetables, herbs, and eggplant to lettuce just before serving.

Pour ¼ cup of the dressing over salad and toss well. Season with salt and pepper. Pass remaining dressing separately.

Eggplant Factoid: Eggplants have a dimple at the blossom end, which can be round or oval in shape. An oval dimple is usually shallower and is often indicative of fewer seeds and a meatier, more desirable eggplant. A deeper, round dimple frequently indicates many seeds inside, especially if the eggplant is large and mature.

Nutrient Analysis: per 1½-cup serving

CALORIES: 111 PROTEIN: 3 grams CARBS.: 16 grams TOTAL FAT: 5 grams SAT. FAT: 1 gram
POLY. FAT: 1 gram MONO. FAT: 3 grams CHOLES.: 0 mg FIBER: 6 grams (Sol. 1 gram)
SODIUM: 18 mgs

Asian Chicken Salad

Crispy slivers of cabbage and crunchy threads of carrot mingle in a tangy peanutty dressing. Grilled chicken makes it a main-course entrée, but the salad can also be served on its own as an Asian coleslaw side dish.

YIELD: ABOUT 2 QUARTS; 6 MAIN-COURSE SALADS
PREPARATION TIME: ABOUT 1 HOUR

Dressing:
⅓ cup olive oil
¼ cup miso (see Notes, page 97)
¼ cup rice wine vinegar
¼ cup soft silken tofu
2 tablespoons fresh lime juice
2 tablespoons sorghum syrup or dark honey
2 tablespoons low-sodium soy sauce
2 tablespoons natural unsweetened peanut butter

2 tablespoons minced green onion (green and white parts)
2 tablespoons pickled ginger (see Notes below)
1½ teaspoons dry mustard
1½ teaspoons minced garlic
1 teaspoon sesame oil

Salad:
8 ounces thinly sliced red cabbage (4 cups)
8 ounces thinly sliced green cabbage (4 cups)
2 medium carrots, cut into julienne strips
1 red bell pepper, cut into thin julienne strips
½ large cucumber, seeded and cut into medium dice
1 pound cooked boneless, skinless chicken, shredded or cut into bite-size
    pieces

Garnish:
3 tablespoons chopped fresh cilantro, without stems
3 tablespoons toasted sesame seeds (see Notes below)

Prepare dressing: Add all ingredients to a blender or food processor and blend until smooth. Set aside. There will be about 2 cups of dressing.

Prepare salad: Combine vegetables and chicken in a large mixing bowl. Add 1 cup dressing and toss well.

Garnish with cilantro and sesame seeds. Pass additional dressing separately.

NOTES: Miso is a fermented soybean paste that is used as a flavoring in Japanese cooking. Its flavor is very concentrated and very salty; use in moderation. It is available at Japanese markets and in the Asian foods section of some supermarkets.

Pickled ginger is a Japanese condiment served with sushi. It is used to cleanse the palate and to enhance flavor. It can be found in the ethnic section of your supermarket or in a Japanese market. If unavailable, you may substitute an equal amount of peeled, minced ginger.

NOTE: To toast sesame seeds, preheat oven to 325 degrees Fahrenheit. Spread seeds on a baking sheet. Bake about 12 minutes, or until seeds are lightly browned and become fragrant. Stir two to three times during baking to ensure even browning. Allow to cool completely before using. Store leftovers, tightly covered, in the refrigerator.

Cabbage Factoid: Cooking, air exposure, and long storage time reduce the vitamin C content of cabbage. This antioxidant is best preserved when cabbage is cut immediately before use.

Nutrient Analysis: per 1 main-course salad

CALORIES: 277   PROTEIN: 30 grams   CARBS.: 16 grams   TOTAL FAT: 10 grams   SAT. FAT: 2 grams

POLY. FAT: 6 grams   MONO. FAT: 2 grams   CHOLES.: 66 mgs   FIBER: 4 grams (Sol. 1 gram)

SODIUM: 505 mgs

Saag Paneer (Creamy Spinach with Peppery Cheese)

Though this classic Indian dish is usually made with spinach, it works well with other greens such as kale. For a less spicy flavor, use plain soy jack cheese.

YIELD: 2 CUPS; 4 (½-CUP) SERVINGS

PREPARATION TIME: 15 MINUTES

1 tablespoon olive oil

1 tablespoon peeled, chopped fresh ginger

1 teaspoon ground coriander

½ teaspoon ground turmeric

½ teaspoon ground cumin

½ teaspoon garam masala or curry powder
1 pound washed, finely chopped fresh spinach leaves or 1 (16-ounce)
   package frozen chopped spinach, thawed and drained
½ teaspoon salt (optional)
3 ounces soy pepper jack cheese, cut into ¼-inch cubes

Heat olive oil in large sauté pan over medium heat. Add ginger and spices and cook, stirring, until mixture is fragrant and begins to bubble, about 30 seconds.

Add spinach and cook over medium-high heat until wilted and tender, about 2 minutes. Turn frequently to ensure even cooking. Season to taste with salt.

Remove from heat and gently stir in cheese. Serve hot.

Spinach Factoid: Researchers are stirring up clues that age-related deficits in memory may be reversed with nutritional interventions of antioxidant-rich foods such as spinach.

Nutrient Analysis: per ½-cup serving
   CALORIES: 124   PROTEIN: 8 grams   CARBS.: 8 grams   TOTAL FAT: 8 grams   SAT. FAT: 1 gram
   POLY. FAT: 1 gram   MONO. FAT: 5 grams   CHOLES.: 0 mg   FIBER: 4 grams   SODIUM: 85 mgs

Curried Creamed Cabbage

Double cooking the cabbage tones down its pungency and brightens its sweetness in this creamy curried sauce. This recipe reflects cabbage's versatility in adapting to a wide range of seasonings.

YIELD: 3 CUPS; 4 (¾-CUP) SERVINGS
PREPARATION TIME: 15 MINUTES

½ head cored, thinly sliced green cabbage (about 1½ pounds)
2 tablespoons olive oil
1½ tablespoons unbleached all-purpose flour
2 teaspoons curry powder
2 tablespoons finely chopped yellow onion
¾ cup unflavored soymilk
Salt and pepper to taste

Cook cabbage in rapidly boiling water for 4 minutes; drain well. Set aside.

Heat oil in a large sauté pan over medium heat and whisk in flour and curry powder to make a smooth paste. Add onion and cook for 1 minute longer. Whisk in soymilk and cook until it thickens slightly. Add cabbage and stir to coat well. Cook just until cabbage is tender, about 2 minutes longer. Season with salt and pepper.

Cabbage Factoid: Cooked cabbage's strong odor comes from its sulfur compounds, which are released into the air during heating.

Nutrient Analysis: per ¾-cup serving
CALORIES: 131   PROTEIN: 5 grams   CARBS.: 16 grams   TOTAL FAT: 7 grams   SAT. FAT: 1 gram
POLY. FAT: 1 gram   MONO. FAT: 4 grams   CHOLES.: 0 mg   FIBER: 6 grams (Sol. 1 gram)   SODIUM: 47 mgs

Crispy Kale Croquettes

Croquettes, the French term for a preparation that is commonly used for potatoes or salmon, means "little crispies." These crunchy pillows are bound with a mildly seasoned cream sauce. Spinach may be substituted. They are a perfect make-ahead side dish.

YIELD: 14 CROQUETTES; 7 (2-CROQUETTE) SERVINGS
PREPARATION TIME: 45 MINUTES

> *1 teaspoon plus 1 tablespoon olive oil*
> *2 bunches kale (about 2 pounds), rinsed and stems and tough ribs*
>   *discarded, or 2 (10-ounce) packages frozen chopped kale, thawed*
>   *and drained*
> *2 tablespoons minced garlic*
> *Salt and pepper to taste*
> *1 tablespoon unbleached all-purpose flour*
> *½ cup unflavored soymilk*
> *1 tablespoon grated Parmesan cheese*
> *Pinch ground nutmeg*
> *Pinch ground cloves*
> *1 cup panko bread crumbs (see Note below)*

Preheat oven to 400 degrees Fahrenheit. Lightly coat a 15 x 10-inch baking sheet with olive oil cooking spray.

Tear kale into bite-size pieces. (If using frozen kale, squeeze thawed kale very dry.)

Heat 1 teaspoon oil in a large nonstick sauté pan over medium-high heat. Add kale and sauté until wilted, about 4 minutes. Add garlic and sauté 1 minute longer. Season with salt and pepper. Drain any excess juices and transfer kale to a medium mixing bowl.

Heat remaining 1 tablespoon olive oil in a 1-quart saucepan over medium heat. Add flour and whisk 1 minute; do not let mixture brown. Gradually add soymilk, whisking until mixture is smooth. Cook until sauce is thick, whisking frequently, about 1 minute. Remove from heat. Add cheese, nutmeg, and cloves. Cool sauce completely.

Spoon sauce over kale; stir to combine. Season with salt and pepper. Mixture should stick together but be dry enough to form croquettes. (If mixture is too wet, you may need to add 1 tablespoon bread crumbs to absorb excess liquid.)

Place bread crumbs on large plate. Using a ⅛-cup scoop or measuring cup for uniformity, form mixture into about 14 marshmallow-size croquettes. Place croquettes on a plate. Carefully roll each croquette in bread crumbs, pressing to adhere. Transfer to another plate. (Can be prepared up to 4 hours ahead.) Cover; chill.

Place croquettes on prepared baking sheet. Coat croquettes generously with a mist of olive oil spray.

Place the baking sheet on the bottom shelf of the oven and bake about 10 minutes. Turn croquettes with a spatula and bake about 15 minutes longer, or until croquettes are light golden.

NOTE: Panko bread crumbs are available in Asian markets or in the ethnic section of your grocery store. Plain dry bread crumbs may be substituted.

Kale Factoid: Recent scientific studies have indicated that, of all the members of the cruciferous vegetable family, kale has the highest content of the antioxidants beta-carotene and vitamin E.

Nutrient Analysis: per 2-croquette serving

CALORIES: 123   PROTEIN: 5 grams   CARBS.: 17 grams   TOTAL FAT: 4 grams   SAT. FAT: 1 gram

POLY. FAT: 1 gram   MONO. FAT: 2 grams   CHOLES.: 1 mg   FIBER: 2 grams (Sol. 1 gram)

SODIUM: 164 mgs

Southern-Style Mustard Greens

Mustard greens have a hint of bitterness that balances nicely with the sweetness in balsamic vinegar. For a milder flavor, include a variety of greens such as Swiss chard or spinach.

YIELD: 2 CUPS; 4 (½-CUP) SERVINGS
PREPARATION TIME: 30 MINUTES

> 1 tablespoon olive oil
> 1 cup chopped red onion
> 1 tablespoon minced garlic
> 1 teaspoon dry mustard powder
> 2 tablespoons balsamic vinegar
> 1 pound clean, chopped fresh mustard greens or other greens (collard, turnip, or beet) or 1 (10-ounce) package frozen chopped mustard greens, thawed and drained
> Salt and pepper to taste

Heat olive oil in a large saucepan or Dutch oven over medium heat. Add onion and cook until wilted and lightly golden, about 6 minutes. Add garlic and mustard powder and cook 1 minute; do not brown garlic.

Add vinegar and mix well. Begin adding the greens, one-third at a time, pressing them down as they begin to wilt.

Reduce heat to medium low and cook, uncovered, until the greens are soft, about 8 minutes. Season with salt and pepper. Serve hot.

Mustard Greens Factoid: Mustard greens are loaded with highly absorbable calcium and vitamins A, C, thiamin, and riboflavin.

Nutrient Analysis: per ½-cup serving

CALORIES: 75 PROTEIN: 4 grams CARBS.: 9 grams TOTAL FAT: 4 grams SAT. FAT: 0 gram

POLY. FAT: 0 gram MONO. FAT: 3 grams CHOLES.: 0 mg FIBER: 5 grams SODIUM: 35 mgs

Nutty Glazed Brussels Sprouts

The nutty taste of Brussels sprouts is enhanced with a pinch of nutmeg, a drizzle of sorghum, and a hint of citrus. The simple elegance of this vegetable dish demands a place for it on your holiday table.

YIELD: 3 CUPS; 4 (¾-CUP) SERVINGS

PREPARATION TIME: 20 MINUTES

1 pound fresh Brussels sprouts or 1 (10-ounce) package frozen Brussels
  sprouts, thawed
2 teaspoons olive oil
Salt and pepper to taste
⅛ teaspoon ground nutmeg
1 teaspoon sorghum syrup or dark honey

Garnish:
1 tablespoon chopped, toasted walnuts (see Note, page 31)
1 teaspoon grated orange peel

Bring 2 quarts salted water to a boil.

Remove outer leaves from sprouts. Trim ends of bases but leave cores intact. Add Brussels sprouts to boiling water and cook until they are fork-tender, about 8 minutes. Drain and immediately transfer to bowl with enough cold water to cover to cool. Quarter each sprout lengthwise. Brussels sprouts can be prepared in advance to this point and refrigerated.

Heat olive oil in a sauté pan over medium-high heat. Sauté Brussels sprouts until they are heated through, about 2 minutes. (It will take slightly longer if Brussels sprouts were cooked and refrigerated in advance.) Season with salt, pepper, and nutmeg. Drizzle sorghum syrup over Brussels sprouts and stir well. Garnish with walnuts and orange peel.

Brussels Sprouts Factoid: Brussels sprouts and cabbage contain a sulfur compound called *sinigrin.* When the vegetable is cut, the sinigrin's by-products emit distinct and pungent flavors. They also possess antibacterial properties.

Nutrient Analysis: per ¾-cup serving

CALORIES: 97   PROTEIN: 4 grams   CARBS.: 15 grams   TOTAL FAT: 4 grams   SAT. FAT: 0.5 gram

POLY. FAT: 1 gram   MONO. FAT: 2 grams   CHOLES.: 0 mg   FIBER: 5 grams (Sol. 2 grams)

SODIUM: 29 mgs

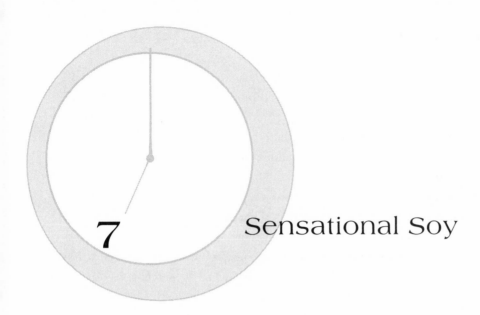

7 Sensational Soy

The longest life spans in the world are found among the people of the Japanese island of Okinawa. It appears they've found a few keys to longevity, and soybeans are an elemental part of their diet. Coincidence? Hardly. There's no doubt they're on to something, and it has everything to do with stopping the clock. Soy has been an integral part of the Asian diet for centuries. Beyond its variety of forms, tastes, and textures, soy products have a multitude of antiaging attributes.

You don't have to resign yourself to a tofu diet to benefit from this metamorphic legume. From a sweet and frosty breakfast smoothie or a rich miso-laced broth to a crisp and tangy stir-fry or a creamy rich dessert, soy has many faces, and its antiaging payoff hits the jackpot.

It's hard to believe that the ubiquitous soybean, now a mainstay in our pantries, was considered another fleeting American fad in the not-so-distant past. Americans still lag behind in global consumption, despite the fact that we produce more than half of the world's soybeans.

There are as many antiaging benefits from soyfoods as there are forms of soyfoods. Let's begin with the phytochemicals. Though most traditional soyfoods are not richly colored by phytochemical pigments, they do have a plethora of one class of phytochemicals called *phytoestrogens*. The predominant forms of these plant estrogens are genistein and daidzein, whose resemblance to human estrogen enables them to simulate some of the hormone's effects on the body.

When introduced in moderation via natural soyfoods, phytoestrogens may provide the essential benefits of human estrogen, with a decreased threat of cancer, through several mechanisms that are not completely understood. Genistein is believed to block a process called *angiogenesis,* or the formation of new blood vessels needed for tumors to grow. Estrogen production declines in postmenopausal women by up to 70 percent, leading to weaker bones and less protection from heart disease and cancer. In men, estrogen levels are significantly lower to begin with, though they do provide a crucial balance to their more dominant hormone, testosterone. With age, male estrogen declines, creating a potential imbalance that may allow a disproportionate testosterone level to hasten the growth of hormonally influenced prostate tumors. But the phytoestrogens in soy appear to slow down or inhibit cancerous cell growth in both men and women.

More is not better when it comes to phytoestrogens, especially isoflavones. This class of phytoestrogens has the greatest capacity to simulate the effects of human estrogen in the body. Extracted or synthesized isoflavones, which are now being added to food through fortification, have hotly contested "benefits." High doses of isoflavones found in products such as powders and pills can be harmful to some people. Mimicking hormones is serious business. Nontraditional soy foods, such as isolated soy proteins and isoflavone supplements, are prime examples of the argument against fortified foods because of the lack of documented evidence in their favor. If in doubt, check with your doctor.

And here's a hot flash on soy: There isn't even a word for this menopausal symptom in the Japanese language. For centuries, Japanese women have enjoyed the beneficial hormonal effects of natural phytoestrogens in soy while minimizing some of the unpleasant symptoms of menopause.

Soy also contains phytosterols, the "cholesterol clone" found in avocados, nuts, seeds, and grains. Phytosterols not only promote heart health, they also may impede cell reproduction in the large intestine, possibly preventing colon cancer. Another phytochemical, phytic acid, is thought to lower cholesterol and may provide protection against some cancers. It may also control blood sugar, cholesterol, and triglycerides. Saponins, yet another phytochemical, may prevent cancer cells from multiplying by interfering with DNA repli-cation. Saponins may also help control blood sugar and lower cholesterol and triglycerides by binding bile acids.

Dr. Mark Messina, an internationally recognized expert on this celebrated legume, maintains that ". . . soyfoods are unique because they are the only foods to provide nutri-tionally relevant amounts of isoflavones. Consuming about two servings of soy per day pro-vides 10 to 15 grams of soy protein and 30 to 50 milligrams of isoflavones. This amount is recommended on a daily basis to derive many of soy's health benefits."

A traditional source of soy protein is the tender green pod known as *edamame* (pro-nounced ed-uh-MAH-may), soybeans that are harvested before they become mature or hard. The young beans nestle in a soft fuzzy pod and have a mild sweet taste. They're a de-licious snack in their unadulterated simplicity and are as pervasive in Japan as pretzels or chips are in the U.S. Requiring little more than a sprinkling of salt, edamame take only five minutes to steam, boil, or microwave. They're eaten like an artichoke leaf, by placing a pod in your mouth and then pulling it out through lightly clenched teeth. The chewy beans are left in your mouth, and the pod is tossed. Or they can be shucked and eaten like peas. A tasty way to jazz them up is with transcontinental Edamame Guacamole and Stop the Clock! Trail Mix.

Left a little longer on the vine, mature soybeans are harvested and dried, much like other dried beans. Whole soybeans are 40 percent protein and an excellent source of fiber. One cup of raw edamame has a whopping 22 grams of protein, while mature soybeans boast 29 grams. In soups or stews, barbecued or refried, prepare soybeans like other dried beans. Though they require soaking for eight hours and a long cooking time, cooked soy-beans are also found in cans for a quicker fix. Unleash the antiaging powers of this sensa-tional legume with Creamy Hummus.

Soymilk is made by cooking ground hulled soybeans with water. The finished prod-uct is filtered and sometimes sweetened. Soymilk is a great alternative to dairy products and provides protein, thiamin, and minerals. Many brands are even fortified with calcium. Low in saturated fat, soymilk is lactose- and cholesterol-free and can replace cow's milk in most recipes. It can be heated or simmered but should not be boiled. Revel in the creamy goodness of soymilk with the satisfying flavors of Chocolate-Caramel Pudding.

Miso is a paste made by cooking and then fermenting soybeans with salt. A variety of grains is sometimes added (e.g., barley, brown rice), and the fermentation period varies, generally from one to three years. All of these options result in a large variety of miso pastes, ranging from mild and yellow to strong and dark brown. In general, the longer the miso is aged, the darker the color and stronger the flavor. Its intensely rich flavor goes a long way to enhance a broth, stew, or marinade. Just a dab is needed.

Where there's fermentation, there are bacteria, and, in this case, fermentation is a good thing. The beneficial bacteria found in unpasteurized miso products are called *probiotics*. Some consider them an aid to improving digestion and the health of the intestinal tract. There is some scientific evidence that fermented products with probiotics can help to prevent some forms of cancer, too. Taste the rich flavors of Grilled Miso Chicken, Miso Rice Porridge, and Miso Soup with Wilted Greens and Roasted Tomatoes.

Tofu is made from cooked soybeans. It is usually purchased in a white block form in textures from soft to extra firm. Tofu is incredibly versatile because it tends to absorb the flavors or seasonings added to the dish in which it's used. Stir-fried, grilled, baked, or raw, explore its chameleon character in Harira with Roasted Vegetables, Banana-Fudge Smoothie, and Old-Fashioned Orange Sherbet.

Creamy Hummus

This creamy Middle Eastern spread takes minutes to prepare and will keep for several days, refrigerated. Serve as an appetizer with warm pita bread cut in bite-size wedges or as a sandwich on warm pita with sliced tomatoes and shredded lettuce.

YIELD: ABOUT 2 CUPS; 8 (¼-CUP) SERVINGS
PREPARATION TIME: 15 MINUTES

1½ cups cooked soybeans or 1 (15-ounce) can, drained and rinsed
1½ cups cooked garbanzo beans or 1 (15-ounce) can, drained and
  rinsed
½ cup warm water
3 tablespoons fresh lime juice
1 tablespoon grated lime peel

1 tablespoon tahini (see Note, page 46)
1½ teaspoons ground cumin
1 teaspoon minced garlic
¾ teaspoon salt
1 tablespoon chopped fresh mint, without stems
1 tablespoon chopped fresh Italian parsley, without stems

Place all ingredients except herbs in the bowl of a food processor or a blender jar. Process or blend until very smooth, about 4 minutes. Transfer to a bowl. Stir in fresh herbs.

Soybean Factoid: The phytoestrogens in soybeans mimic hormones and fight some of the symptoms of PMS and menopause.

Nutrient Analysis: per ¼-cup serving

CALORIES: 117   PROTEIN: 9 grams   CARBS.: 12 grams   TOTAL FAT: 5 grams   SAT. FAT: 1 gram
POLY. FAT: 2 grams   MONO. FAT: 1 gram   CHOLES.: 0 mg   FIBER: 4 grams (Sol. 0.8 gram)
SODIUM: 222 mgs

Edamame Guacamole

This delicious imposter has 30 percent fewer calories and fat than traditional guacamole, plus more protein, greater nutrient diversity, and lots of isoflavones.

YIELD: 2 CUPS; 16 (2-TABLESPOON) SERVINGS
PREPARATION TIME: 15 MINUTES

1 cup shelled edamame (about 12 ounces unshelled)
½ cup unflavored soymilk
2 tablespoons chopped fresh cilantro, without stems

2 minced garlic cloves
1 teaspoon chopped chipotle chiles (optional; see Note, page 63)
1 large ripe avocado
2 teaspoons fresh lime juice
Salt and pepper to taste

Garnish:
1 tablespoon chopped fresh cilantro, without stems

Cook edamame in salted boiling water for 5 minutes. Drain and cool to room temperature.

Combine edamame, soymilk, cilantro, garlic, and chiles (if using) in the bowl of a food processor. Process until mixture is very smooth, about 3 minutes. Set aside.

Peel and pit avocado and place in a medium mixing bowl. Add lime juice and mash with a fork, leaving small chunks. Add edamame mixture and stir just to combine. Season with salt and pepper. Garnish with cilantro.

Edamame Factoid: In addition to being a great snack, 1 cup of cooked edamame has 7 grams of fiber and a whopping 22 grams of protein.

Nutrient Analysis: per 2-tablespoon serving

CALORIES: 45   PROTEIN: 3 grams   CARBS.: 3 grams   TOTAL FAT: 3 grams   SAT. FAT: 0.5 gram

POLY. FAT: 1 gram   MONO. FAT: 0 gram   CHOLES.: 0 mg   FIBER: 2 grams   SODIUM: 5 mgs

Stop the Clock! Trail Mix

This rendition of trail mix is loaded with fiber and protein. Make this nutrient-dense recipe your own by adding your favorite dried fruits or seeds.

YIELD: ABOUT 6 CUPS; 18 (⅓-CUP) SERVINGS

PREPARATION TIME: 5 MINUTES

> *3 cups unsalted soynuts (see Note below)*
> *1 cup dried cranberries*
> *1 cup dried blueberries*
> *1 cup Stop the Clock! Grainola (page 157) or 1 cup granola*

Place soynuts in a medium mixing bowl. Add berries and Grainola. Stir to combine. Store in an airtight container for up to 2 weeks.

NOTE: Soynuts are roasted soybeans and can be found in most health food stores and supermarkets.

Soy Factoid: Not only is the high-calorie, top-protein soybean a key energy source for humans, but the oil of this versatile bean is used to produce biodiesel to fuel engines.

Nutrient Analysis: per ⅓-cup serving

CALORIES: 192   PROTEIN: 10 grams   CARBS.: 23 grams   TOTAL FAT: 7 grams   SAT. FAT: 1 gram
POLY. FAT: 4 grams   MONO. FAT: 2 grams   CHOLES.: 0 mg   FIBER: 7 grams   SODIUM: 1 mg

Miso Soup with Wilted Greens and Roasted Tomatoes

In Japan, miso soup is an indispensable part of breakfast. This heartier version is an easy way to enjoy miso's rich flavors and restorative powers throughout the day.

YIELD: 6 CUPS; 4 (1½-CUP) SERVINGS
PREPARATION TIME: 30 MINUTES

3 unpeeled garlic cloves
5 plum tomatoes (about 1 pound)
1 tablespoon olive oil
¾ cup finely chopped yellow onion
1 tablespoon peeled, finely chopped fresh ginger
4 cups fat-free, low-sodium chicken or vegetable broth
2 tablespoons sweet white miso (see Note, page 97)
4 ounces firm tofu, drained and cut into ¼-inch dice
1 cup fresh spinach leaves, cut in fine chiffonade (see Note, page 61)

Garnish:
1 very thinly sliced green onion (green and white parts)

Preheat oven to 450 degrees Fahrenheit. Lightly coat a 15 x 10-inch baking sheet with olive oil cooking spray. Wrap garlic cloves in small piece of aluminum foil; seal tightly. Cut tomatoes crosswise into ½-inch-thick slices and arrange in a single layer on the baking sheet.

Place foil-wrapped garlic on the baking sheet with the tomatoes. Roast garlic and tomatoes in oven, switching position of pan halfway through roasting, about 35 minutes total, or until garlic is tender and tomatoes are lightly charred. Unwrap garlic, cool slightly, and remove skin. Add garlic and tomatoes to a food processor or blender and purée. Set aside.

Heat olive oil in a 2-quart saucepan over medium heat. Add onion and sauté until just starting to brown, about 8 minutes. Add ginger and sauté for 1 minute. Add broth and puréed tomatoes and bring to a boil. Whisk in miso until it has dissolved in soup. Add tofu and spinach and simmer 1 minute.

Serve warm, garnished with green onion.

> *Miso Factoid:* Nonpasteurized miso not only contains beneficial bacteria and their enzymes (probiotics), it also contains richer flavors and aromas that are lost in the process of pasteurization.

Nutrient Analysis: per 1½-cup serving

CALORIES: 145   PROTEIN: 12 grams   CARBS.: 13 grams   TOTAL FAT: 6 grams   SAT. FAT: 1 gram
POLY. FAT: 1 gram   MONO. FAT: 3 grams   CHOLES.: 0 mg   FIBER: 3 grams (Sol. 1 gram)
SODIUM: 313 mgs

Grilled Miso Chicken

The tangy marinade used in this recipe can be prepared in minutes. It's a simple way to impart tantalizing flavors to fish or tofu as well. Be sure to use the light miso, because the darker paste is salty and can be overpowering when combined with other seasonings.

YIELD: 4 SERVINGS

PREPARATION TIME: 30 MINUTES PLUS 1 HOUR MARINATING TIME

1 tablespoon light soy sauce
¼ cup mirin or sake
1 tablespoon light miso (see Note, page 109)
1 tablespoon tahini (see Note, page 46)
1 finely chopped green onion (white and green parts)

1 tablespoon chopped fresh cilantro, without stems
1 tablespoon peeled, minced fresh ginger
1 teaspoon minced garlic
1 pound boneless, skinless chicken breasts

Garnish:
2 tablespoons chopped fresh cilantro, without stems
1 teaspoon toasted sesame seeds (see Note, page 98)

Prepare marinade: Combine soy sauce, mirin, miso, tahini, green onion, cilantro, ginger, and garlic in a medium mixing bowl. This will yield about ½ cup of marinade. Coat chicken with mixture and marinate for a minimum of 1 hour or refrigerate overnight, turning several times.

Preheat outdoor grill or broiler to medium-high heat. Remove chicken from marinade and transfer marinade to a small saucepan over medium heat. Bring just to a boil, reduce heat, and let simmer.

Blot excess marinade from chicken to prevent burning. Place chicken on grill and baste with the cooked marinade during cooking. Cook chicken about 3 minutes per side, depending on thickness, or until juices run clear.

Garnish with cilantro and sesame seeds.

Miso Factoid: Miso is high in sodium and should be used sparingly. It is a great substitute for salt or soy sauce in many recipes.

Nutrient Analysis: per serving
CALORIES: 182   PROTEIN: 28 grams   CARBS.: 4 grams   TOTAL FAT: 4 grams   SAT. FAT: 1 gram
POLY. FAT: 1 gram   MONO. FAT: 1 gram   CHOLES.: 66 mgs   FIBER: 1 gram   SODIUM: 327 mgs

Harira with Roasted Vegetables

Harira, a hearty and satisfying stew, is traditionally served to break the fast at the end of Ramadan, the ninth month of the Muslim calendar. This vegetarian version is loaded with fiber. It is thickened with the starch of garbanzo beans and lentils. Roasting some of the vegetables instead of cooking them in the stew gives an added flavor dimension.

YIELD: 2 QUARTS; 8 (1-CUP) SERVINGS
PREPARATION TIME: 1 HOUR

> ½ pound firm tofu
> 1 medium peeled yellow onion, halved and then quartered
> 1 (8-inch) stalk celery, quartered crosswise
> 1 tablespoon extra-virgin olive oil
> 1 tablespoon minced garlic
> 2 teaspoons ground cumin
> ½ teaspoon ground turmeric
> ½ teaspoon ground cardamom
> ½ teaspoon ground cinnamon
> ½ teaspoon ground white pepper
> 4 cups fat-free chicken or vegetable broth
> 1½ cups cooked garbanzo beans or 1 (15-ounce) can, rinsed and drained
> ½ cup dry lentils, rinsed and drained
> 1 cup tomatoes peeled, halved, seeded, chopped or 1 cup tomato sauce
>   (see Note, page 195)
> Salt and pepper to taste
>
> **Garnish:**
> ¼ cup finely chopped fresh cilantro, without stems

Wrap tofu block in paper towels or a cotton towel and place a heavy weight, such as a heavy skillet, on top. Let stand 30 minutes to release excess water. Cut into ½-inch dice.

Preheat oven to 425 degrees Fahrenheit. Lightly coat a 15 x 10-inch baking sheet with olive oil cooking spray. Place quartered onion and celery on baking sheet and roast about 25 minutes or until golden brown. Cool and finely chop the onion and the celery.

Heat olive oil in a large sauté pan over medium heat. Add onion, celery, garlic, and spices. Cook, stirring, until the spices are fragrant, about 2 minutes. Add broth and bring to a boil. Add garbanzo beans, lentils, and tomatoes, and simmer about 30 minutes or until lentils are nearly tender. Add diced tofu and simmer 15 minutes.

Season with salt and pepper and garnish with cilantro.

NOTE: If reheating soup the second day, you may need to thin it with additional broth, readjust the seasoning, and add more fresh cilantro.

Soybean Factoid: Soybeans contain an antidisease agent called *genistein,* which has been shown to interfere with cancer growth at virtually every stage.

Nutrient Analysis: per 1-cup serving

CALORIES: 203   PROTEIN: 13 grams   CARBS.: 27 grams   TOTAL FAT: 5 grams   SAT. FAT: 1 gram
POLY. FAT: 2 grams   MONO. FAT: 2 grams   CHOLES.: 0 mg   FIBER: 8 grams (Sol. 2 grams)
SODIUM: 99 mgs

Miso Rice Porridge

Rice porridge is a mainstay of the Asian diet. Known as "congee" in China, it's called "okayu" in Japan. The rice is cooked in twice the usual liquid measure, resulting in a thick brothy gruel. Slow simmering in soymilk instead of water adds a nutty flavor and lots of protein. The saltiness of miso and the sweetness of sorghum syrup and ginger yield a surprisingly delicious balance of flavors.

YIELD: 3 CUPS; 4 (¾-CUP) SERVINGS

PREPARATION TIME: 50 MINUTES

> ½ cup long-grain brown rice
> 2½ cups unflavored soymilk
> 1½ tablespoons light yellow miso paste
> 2 tablespoons sorghum syrup or dark honey
> 1 tablespoon minced crystallized ginger (see Note below)

Rinse rice and place in a 3-quart saucepan to prevent boiling over. Add soymilk and bring almost to a boil. (Soymilk should only be simmered, as boiling can cause it to curdle.) Reduce heat, cover, and simmer for 50 minutes. There will be excess liquid.

Remove from heat and stir in remaining ingredients. Serve hot.

NOTE: The acids in fresh ginger can cause the milk to break or curdle. If crystallized ginger is not available, use 1 teaspoon dried ginger.

Miso Factoid: One tablespoon of miso has 2 grams of protein.

Nutrient Analysis: per ¾-cup serving

CALORIES: 177   PROTEIN: 7 grams   CARBS.: 29 grams   TOTAL FAT: 4 grams   SAT. FAT: 0.5 gram

POLY. FAT: 2 grams   MONO. FAT: 1 gram   CHOLES.: 0 mg   FIBER: 3 grams   SODIUM: 298 mgs

Old-Fashioned Orange Sherbet

This frosty and luscious concoction is flavored with fruit juices. Sherbet is distinct from sorbet in that it sometimes, but not always, contains milk. Orange juice concentrate is used in this recipe to intensify the flavor without adding additional sweeteners. Garnish with mixed berries for a refreshing dessert or snack.

YIELD: 3 CUPS; 4 (¾-CUP) SERVINGS
PREPARATION TIME: 30 MINUTES

> 2 cups vanilla soymilk
> 6 ounces frozen organic orange juice concentrate
> ½ cup silken tofu
> 1 tablespoon fresh lime juice
> 1 teaspoon grated orange peel (or lime peel)
> ½ teaspoon pure vanilla extract
> 1 tablespoon sorghum syrup or dark honey

Combine all ingredients in the bowl of a food processor or a blender jar. Process until combined. Chill mixture for 30 minutes.

Freeze sherbet according to the manufacturer's instructions for your ice cream maker. If you do not have an ice cream maker, place the mixture in a medium mixing bowl and place in the freezer. Freeze until partially frozen, about 1 hour. Remove mixture from the freezer and mix well with a hand mixer or pulse with a food processor to break up ice crystals. Repeat freezing and mixing steps one or two times.

Soy Factoid: The phytoestrogens in soy help retain bone mass and reduce the risk for osteoporosis.

Nutrient Analysis: per ¾-cup serving

CALORIES: 128   PROTEIN: 7 grams   CARBS.: 19 grams   TOTAL FAT: 3 grams   SAT. FAT: 0 gram

POLY. FAT: 1 gram   MONO. FAT: 1 gram   CHOLES.: 0 mg   FIBER: 2 grams   SODIUM: 36 mgs

Chocolate-Caramel Pudding

Creamy and smooth, chocolaty and not too sweet, this ultimate comfort food can satisfy a midday sweet tooth or finish a fabulous meal. Served warm or cold, this silky crowd pleaser takes just minutes to prepare.

YIELD: 2 CUPS; 4 (½-CUP) SERVINGS

PREPARATION TIME: 10 MINUTES

¼ cup unsweetened natural cocoa powder
¼ cup cornstarch
¼ teaspoon salt
2 cups unflavored soymilk
½ cup sorghum syrup
2 teaspoons pure vanilla extract

Combine cocoa powder, cornstarch, and salt in a 1-quart saucepan. Add just enough of the soymilk to make a smooth paste. Gradually stir in remaining soymilk and sorghum syrup.

Cook over medium heat, stirring constantly, until mixture begins to thicken. Remove from heat and stir in vanilla. Pour into four serving dishes and chill.

Soy Factoid: Soymilk is a highly nutritious beverage that is available worldwide. It can usually be substituted for cow's milk in most recipes.

Nutrient Analysis: per ½-cup serving

CALORIES: 213   PROTEIN: 5 grams   CARBS.: 43 grams   TOTAL FAT: 3 grams   SAT. FAT: 1 gram

POLY. FAT: 1 gram   MONO. FAT: 1 gram   CHOLES.: 0 mg   FIBER: 3 grams   SODIUM: 165 mgs

Banana-Fudge Smoothie

Creamy and delicious, this smoothie is great for breakfast or a midday pick-me-up.

YIELD: 3 CUPS; 2 (1½-CUP) SERVINGS

PREPARATION TIME: 5 MINUTES

1½ cups very cold vanilla soymilk
½ cup soft silken tofu
2 ripe medium bananas, frozen and cut into 1-inch chunks
2 tablespoons unsweetened natural cocoa powder
1 teaspoon sorghum syrup or dark honey

Combine all ingredients in the bowl of a food processor or blender jar. Blend until smooth. Pour into glasses and serve immediately.

Soy Factoid: Soy protein is easier for the kidneys to process than animal protein. This may reduce the risk of certain kidney problems.

Nutrient Analysis: per 1½-cup serving

CALORIES: 247   PROTEIN: 10 grams   CARBS.: 48 grams   TOTAL FAT: 4 grams   SAT. FAT: 1 gram

POLY. FAT: 0 gram   MONO. FAT: 2 grams   CHOLES.: 0 mg   FIBER: 4 grams   SODIUM: 18 mgs

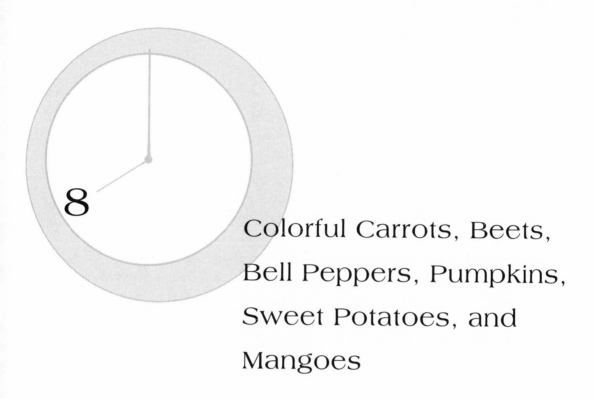

8

Colorful Carrots, Beets, Bell Peppers, Pumpkins, Sweet Potatoes, and Mangoes

Crimson red, fiery orange, brilliant yellow—the confluence of these vibrant colors is a feast for more than our eyes. These lush pigments render a lavish profusion of antiaging utility in the form of beta-carotene and vitamin C. In addition to the overall antioxidant protection they confer, they bolster immunity and fight cancer.

CARROTS

Shortages of everyday commodities pinched the pantries of millions of kitchens during World War II. Cooks on both sides of the Atlantic tested their creative mettle to find substitutes for baking supplies such as butter and eggs. To solve the shortage, an unimposing candidate stepped forward, the carrot. Its sweet moisture lent tenderness to the crumb of what has become a classic dessert. Dense and spicy, carrot cake's rich flavors are steeped in tradition. This breakout role for a humble root vegetable led to its star status and universal recognition.

Versatile, economical, and accessible, carrots process sweet, unassertive flavors that evoke simplicity and freshness, but their bold and vibrant color screams "stop the clock!" Carrots and their like-hued counterparts are antioxidant gold mines. They contain phenolic compounds and boatloads of beta-carotene, a combo believed to reduce the risk of several cancers and to provide protection against heart disease and memory loss.

Peels intact and lightly cooked are the routes to the carrot's optimal offerings. Like the tomato, the heating process releases the carrot's vitamins, making them easier for our bodies to absorb. One of the carrot's antiaging properties is its ability to scavenge free radicals to maintain oxidative balance. Other benefits derive from beta-carotene's conversion to vitamin A and the collective impact of its components on promoting keen vision.

Though preformed vitamin A is available from sources such as meat, liver, and eggs, there are many reasons to limit our intake of animal products due to their high levels of saturated fats and cholesterol. In addition, excess intake of vitamin A from supplements can be harmful. Another way to get your vitamin A is from its precursors, which are found in plant foods. The carrot's orange pigments, called *carotenoids,* are precursors that convert to vitamin A in the body. It's true that your skin can turn orange if you eat too many carrots, but you can't overdose on them. And a faux tan pales in comparison to the toxic repercussions of excess vitamin A.

Besides, carrots aren't the only way to carotene. Creamy pumpkin, delectable mango, crunchy red bell pepper, and the succulent sweet potato offer a diverse selection and plenty of creative rein to meet your antioxidant quota. But first, consider all of the carrot's possibilities. Tender coins float in a creamy dill sauce. Crunchy threads and plump raisins glisten in tangy ginger vinaigrette. Bright, perky baby carrots are ideal for snacking. The world over, carrots are loved and reinvented daily. You can taste the distant flavors of India in Bengali Carrot Sauté and Panch Puran.

BEETS

Another unsung hero is the beet, considered the sweetest of all vegetables. The bravado of its color and its sweet earthy flavor complement a diverse range of dishes and cuisines. And beneath its bold exterior is an antiaging powerhouse. Beets are a rich reserve of betaine, a life-promoting substance that supports liver function and optimizes its detoxification capacity. Betaine also appears to suppress levels of a potentially harmful amino acid—homocysteine, a pro-oxidant associated with promoting heart disease.

Beet roots are also a stellar source of *pectin,* a soluble fiber. This form of fiber is believed to lower blood cholesterol by binding it and thus decreasing the amount absorbed by the body. Pectin also attracts water and turns into a gel, thus slowing digestion. This is beneficial in the case of diabetes because it slows the rise in blood sugar after eating. Pectin's actions also slow digestion, promoting satiety while decreasing hunger.

Many of us forget about the riches nestled in a beet's crispy top. Like other dark leafy vegetables, beet greens are loaded with carotenoids. Their chlorophyll-tinted green belies their abundance of carotenoids, typically linked with golden-yellow colors. And these tasty greens are packed with folate and B vitamins. Perfect for juicing or salads, they can be prepared like any other leafy greens. Unearth the treasures of this hardy root vegetable, and relish it from top to bottom in Moroccan Beet Salad.

BELL PEPPERS

Bell peppers are an excellent source of vitamin C. The shiny red bell pepper lounges on the vine longer than its green sibling, soaking up more sunlight, intensifying its vibrant color, boosting its reserve of carotenoids, and imparting sun-drenched sweetness. The red bell is a pillar of antioxidant strength. Turn up the heat on this sweet mild pepper and simmer a batch of Red Pepper Confit and Roasted Pepper Soup.

PUMPKINS

The lively carotenoid family also colors the fiery pumpkin. Though most edible varieties wind up in pies on Thanksgiving, the pumpkin has incredible culinary versatility to bolster your antiaging armada. This time-honored vegetable is one of the hardiest staples of the global pantry. It is loaded with carotenoids, potassium, and vitamin C.

Give your transmission a kick start with a steaming bowl of Casey's Pumpkin Soup or a dollop of creamy Pumpkin Butter.

SWEET POTATOES

The sweet potato is another fall favorite with a nutrient profile similar to that of the pumpkin. It has the added *oomph* of *alpha-tocopherol,* the plant form of vitamin E, another antioxidant. Whether enjoyed as a starch, in a pie, or in a salad, the sweet potato is usually eaten without the peel. But, as with many of the other antiaging foods, its optimal benefits are observed with the peel intact. Boil it, roast it, or bake it, but remove the skin *after* cooking to maximize its virile powers.

Tock tick, turn back the clock with the homespun flavors of Roasted Sweet Potatoes with Rosemary or Caribbean Sweet Potatoes.

MANGOES

A trip to nirvana is just a bite away with the mango. Peel back its burnished exterior, and the sunburst colors of this fruit beckon with creamy sweetness. Once a tropical rarity, the mainstream mango is savored in smoothies, sorbets, chutneys, and salsas. A true aficionado prefers it plain, maybe with a squeeze of lime, in its unadulterated glory.

But can a fruit of such indulgence possess antiaging powers? A resounding yes! The torrid hue of a ripe mango is attributable to our now familiar carotenoids as well as something called *violaxanthin,* which holds promise as a cancer-fighting commando.

Mangoes thrive in sultry climates and yield high concentrations of phytochemicals, which increase during ripening. As with overconsumption of carrots, gorging on mangoes can result in a yellow tinge to the skin due to carotenemia. Mangoes are also high in sugar, so try to restrain yourself. Though many Asian recipes prize the unripened green mango for pickles and salads, its nutritional profile is not the same, and in some cases, it's a different mango altogether. Taste the tropics with a prescription from paradise. Sip your way to youth with a Sweet Mango Lassi.

Roasted Pepper Soup

This thick, smoky-flavored soup can be prepared in advance and also freezes well. For an extra zing, add a little hot chile to the mix.

YIELD: 1¼ QUARTS; 4 (1¼-CUP) SERVINGS
PREPARATION TIME: 30 MINUTES

> *2 medium red bell peppers*
> *1 tablespoon olive oil*
> *1 cup chopped red onion*
> *½ teaspoon ground cumin*
> *1 teaspoon ground coriander*
> *¼ teaspoon ground cinnamon*
> *1 tablespoon chopped fresh oregano or 1 teaspoon dried*
> *2 medium (about ½ pound) peeled, halved, seeded, chopped tomatoes*
> *   (see Note, page 195) or 1 cup tomato sauce*
> *3 cups fat-free chicken or vegetable broth*
> *Salt and pepper to taste*

Garnish:
2 tablespoons chopped fresh cilantro, without stems

Roast the whole bell peppers under a broiler or on the stovetop, turning occasionally until the skin blisters and chars all over. Place in a bowl, cover with a lid, and let steam to loosen the skins. Carefully peel away skins and remove seeds. Cut peppers into medium dice. Set aside.

Heat olive oil in a 3-quart saucepan over medium heat. Add onion and sauté until it just begins to brown, about 6 minutes. Reduce heat to low and add the bell peppers, cumin, coriander, cinnamon, and oregano. Cook, stirring constantly, until fragrant, about 1 minute.

Carefully add tomatoes and broth. Bring mixture to a boil, reduce heat to low, and simmer for 5 minutes. Carefully transfer hot soup to the bowl of a food processor or a blender jar. Process until smooth. Season with salt and pepper.

Serve immediately, garnished with cilantro.

Oregano Factoid: Oregano and other herbs such as thyme, dill, and rosemary have powerful antioxidant action. Oregano is also prized for its antiseptic properties, and its extract is used in many mouthwashes.

Nutrient Analysis: per 1¼-cup serving

CALORIES: 102   PROTEIN: 6 grams   CARBS.: 12 grams   TOTAL FAT: 4 grams   SAT. FAT: 0.5 gram

POLY. FAT: 0 gram   MONO. FAT: 3 grams   CHOLES.: 0 mg   FIBER: 3 grams (Sol. 1 gram)

SODIUM: 136 mgs

Casey's Pumpkin Soup

Casey Hayden, acclaimed Spago alum, has an eponymous hot spot, Casey's Bakery and Café, in Sacramento, California. When the temperatures plummet in the fall, his popular pumpkin soup sells especially well. It's a great make-ahead starter for Thanksgiving dinner and makes an everyday meal special.

YIELD: 1¼ QUARTS; 4 (1¼-CUP) SERVINGS

PREPARATION TIME: 15 MINUTES

1 medium red bell pepper
1 tablespoon olive oil
1 medium finely chopped red onion
½ teaspoon ground cumin
½ teaspoon ground nutmeg

2 cups fat-free chicken or vegetable broth
1¾ cups pumpkin purée (15 ounces)
1 cup unflavored soymilk
Salt and pepper to taste

Roast the whole bell pepper under a broiler or on the stovetop, turning occasionally, until the skin blisters and chars all over. Place in a bowl, cover with a lid, and let steam to loosen the skin. Carefully peel away skin and remove seeds. Cut pepper into medium dice. Set aside.

Heat oil in a 3-quart saucepan over medium heat. Add onion and bell pepper and sauté until onion is softened but not browned, about 5 minutes. Add spices and cook until fragrant, about 1 minute.

Carefully add broth and pumpkin and bring to a boil. Reduce heat to low and simmer about 8 minutes. Cool slightly.

Transfer soup mixture to a blender jar or the bowl of a food processor. Carefully blend or process the hot soup mixture until smooth.

Return soup to pan. Add soymilk and heat until hot; do not boil. Season with salt and pepper.

Pumpkin Factoid: A dark, antioxidant-rich oil is pressed from the dried seeds of certain varieties of pumpkin. This pumpkin seed oil is rich in vitamins and omega fatty acids. It should not be heated but adds a distinctive, nutty flavor when added to salad dressings.

Nutrient Analysis: per 1¼-cup serving

CALORIES: 123   PROTEIN: 7 grams   CARBS.: 14 grams   TOTAL FAT: 5 grams   SAT. FAT: 1 gram
POLY. FAT: 1 gram   MONO. FAT: 3 grams   CHOLES.: 0 mg   FIBER: 6 grams (Sol. 1 gram)
SODIUM: 100 mgs

Moroccan Beet Salad

Don't toss the beet tops! This flavorful salad combines the nutritious greens with tender beets and Middle Eastern seasonings.

YIELD: 1½ QUARTS; 8 (¾-CUP) SERVINGS
PREPARATION TIME: 1 HOUR

Dressing:
⅓ *cup extra-virgin olive oil*
¼ *cup red wine vinegar or balsamic vinegar*
1 tablespoon sorghum syrup or dark honey
1 tablespoon Dijon mustard
1 tablespoon ground cumin
1 teaspoon ground coriander
1 teaspoon ground turmeric
½ *teaspoon ground cardamom*
½ *teaspoon ground cinnamon*
Salt to taste

Salad:
8 medium-large beets (about 2 pounds) with green tops
1 cup peeled, halved, seeded, chopped tomatoes (see Note, page 195)
Salt and pepper to taste

Garnish:
¼ *cup chopped fresh cilantro, without stems*

Prepare dressing: Combine all ingredients in a large bowl and whisk until thoroughly combined. Makes about ¾ cup dressing.

Prepare salad: Wash beets well, being careful not to break their skins. Cut off the tops, leaving a stalk of about 1½ inches. Reserve green tops and set aside. Place beets in a 3-quart saucepan, cover with cold water, and bring to a boil. Reduce heat to medium, cover, and cook until a knife can be easily inserted and removed, about 30 minutes. Remove from heat and allow to cool in cooking water. Slip off the beet skins, trim off the tops, and cut beets into bite-size pieces. Toss beets and tomatoes with ¼ cup of the dressing. Set aside to marinate.

Wash greens. Transfer greens, with some water still clinging to the leaves, to a large pot over high heat. Cook, stirring, until just wilted but still bright green, about 4 minutes. Drain greens; squeeze out excess moisture. Cool slightly; chop coarsely.

Transfer greens to a medium bowl. Add 1 tablespoon of the dressing and toss to coat. Season greens with salt and pepper. Arrange tomatoes and beets in the center of a platter and surround with greens. Garnish with cilantro. Pass remaining dressing separately.

Beet Factoid: The beet greens have twice as much potassium as the beets themselves, and they are loaded with the antioxidant beta-carotene. Some studies have shown that they contain a compound that suppresses cravings for nicotine, thus aiding smokers to kick the urge to smoke.

Nutrient Analysis: per ¾-cup serving
CALORIES: 93   PROTEIN: 3 grams   CARBS.: 13 grams   TOTAL FAT: 4 grams   SAT. FAT: 1 gram
POLY. FAT: 0 gram   MONO. FAT: 3 grams   CHOLES.: 0 mg   FIBER: 4 grams (Sol. 1 gram)
SODIUM: 183 mgs

Salade Romesco

Romesco is a classic Spanish sauce with a myriad of variations, usually served on bread or pasta. The primary ingredients are dried chiles, almonds, olive oil, garlic, and sometimes tomatoes or roasted red bell peppers. This recipe converts the classic sauce to a vinaigrette by staying true to the ingredients but tweaking the proportions with more vinegar and less oil. Wonderful on crisp baby greens, the dressing is delicious as a sauce or dip for roasted or grilled vegetables.

YIELD: 6 SERVINGS

PREPARATION TIME: 40 MINUTES

Dressing:
1 medium red bell pepper
¼ cup toasted almonds (see Note, page 133)
1 teaspoon chopped canned chipotle chiles (see Note, page 63)
3 peeled garlic cloves
1 teaspoon grated lemon peel
¼ cup red wine vinegar or balsamic vinegar
⅓ cup extra-virgin olive oil
Salt and pepper to taste

Salad:
6 cups baby spinach, rinsed and dried
1½ cups (about 8 ounces) cherry tomatoes, quartered
1 cup seeded, diced cucumber
¼ cup pitted, sliced kalamata olives
1 tablespoon finely chopped fresh oregano
1 tablespoon finely chopped fresh mint leaves, without stems
Salt and pepper to taste

Prepare dressing: Roast whole bell pepper under a broiler or on the stovetop, turning occasionally until skin blisters and chars all over. Place in a bowl, cover with a lid, and let steam to loosen the skin. Carefully peel skin and remove seeds. Cut pepper into medium dice and place in the bowl of a food processor or blender jar.

Add almonds, chiles, garlic, lemon peel, and vinegar. Process until smooth. With the machine running, add the olive oil in a thin stream through the feed tube; the sauce will thicken. Season with salt and pepper. There will be about 1 cup of dressing.

Prepare salad: Combine all salad ingredients except seasoning in a large mixing bowl. Pour 3 tablespoons of the dressing over salad and toss well. Season with salt and pepper. Serve immediately. Pass extra dressing.

NOTE: To toast almonds, spread nuts on an ungreased sheet pan. Bake in a preheated 350-degree Fahrenheit oven about 6 minutes, stirring occasionally, or until golden brown.

Bell Pepper Factoid: Green bell peppers are the most common type and are usually less expensive. Red and yellow peppers stay on the vine longer, yielding more flavor and commanding a higher price. No matter which color you favor, they're all rich sources of vitamin C.

Nutrient Analysis: per serving

CALORIES: 85   PROTEIN: 3 grams   CARBS.: 7 grams   TOTAL FAT: 6 grams   SAT. FAT: 1 gram
POLY. FAT: 1 gram   MONO. FAT: 4 grams   CHOLES.: 0 mg   FIBER: 3 grams (Sol. 1 gram)
SODIUM: 116 mgs

Bengali Carrot Sauté

The Bengal area of India boasts a distinctively flavorful cuisine. *Panch Puran* (see page 135) is a regional seasoning that combines equal parts of five indigenous spices. This spice blend is often roasted or fried before use to release the full flavors of the whole seeds it contains.

Add it to everything from chutneys and curries to fried potatoes. David McMillan, an award-winning chef in Dallas, shares his recipe, which uses spices that can be found in most grocery stores.

YIELD: 2 CUPS; 4 (½-CUP) SERVINGS
PREPARATION TIME: 15 MINUTES

> *4 medium peeled carrots (about 12 ounces), thinly sliced on the*
>   *diagonal*
> *2 tablespoons extra-virgin olive oil*
> *2 teaspoons* Panch Puran *(see Note below)*
> *1 tablespoon sorghum syrup or dark honey*
> *1½ tablespoons chopped fresh cilantro, without stems*

Cook carrots in a pot of boiling salted water until crisp-tender, about 1 minute. Drain and rinse under cold water.

Heat oil in a sauté pan over medium heat. Add *Panch Puran* and swirl pan until spices are fragrant and just beginning to pop, about 30 seconds. Stir in carrots and heat through. Drizzle with sorghum syrup. Stir well and sprinkle with cilantro.

NOTE: Substitute 1 teaspoon garam masala or curry powder for *Panch Puran* if desired.

Carrot Factoid: Cooking carrots will not decrease their content of the antioxidant beta-carotene. Recent studies indicate that cooking may *increase* its availability by softening the plant tissue and allowing greater release of the substance.

Nutrient Analysis: per ½-cup serving
CALORIES: 97   PROTEIN: 1 gram   CARBS.: 15 grams   TOTAL FAT: 4 grams   SAT. FAT: 1 gram
POLY. FAT: 0 gram   MONO. FAT: 2 grams   CHOLES.: 0 mg   FIBER: 3 grams (Sol. 1 gram)
SODIUM: 27 mgs

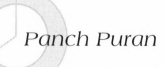

Panch Puran

Yield: ½ cup

 ¼ cup whole fennel seeds
 1 tablespoon white sesame seeds
 1 tablespoon whole yellow mustard seeds
 1 tablespoon whole coriander seeds
 1 tablespoon crushed cardamom seeds

Combine seeds and store in an airtight container.

Caribbean Sweet Potatoes

These creamy golden spuds deserve a place on the table with regularity, not just on Thanksgiving.

Yield: 2 cups; 4 (½-cup) servings
Preparation time: 90 minutes

 1½ pounds sweet potatoes
 3 tablespoons olive oil
 ½ cup unflavored soymilk
 1½ teaspoons salt
 ½ teaspoon ground cinnamon
 ¼ teaspoon ground ginger
 ⅛ teaspoon ground nutmeg

Preheat oven to 400 degrees Fahrenheit. Scrub sweet potatoes and pierce them in several places with the tines of a fork. Place them directly on an oven rack and bake 50 to 60 minutes, or until very tender when pierced with a fork. Remove from oven and cool.

Reduce the oven temperature to 375 degrees Fahrenheit. Lightly coat a shallow 1-quart baking dish with olive oil cooking spray.

When cool enough to handle, scoop sweet potatoes from their skins and mash or rice them in a large bowl. Mix in the oil, soymilk, salt, and spices. Spoon sweet potatoes into prepared dish. (The recipe can be made to this point a day ahead and refrigerated. Let it return to room temperature before proceeding.) Bake about 30 minutes, or until heated through and bubbly.

Sweet Potato Factoid: Sweet potatoes are not the same as yams. Sweet potatoes, unlike yams, are grown in the United States and are sweeter and more moist. Nutritionally speaking, sweet potatoes are higher in the antioxidant vitamins—C, E, and especially A. Yams contain virtually no vitamin A.

Nutrient Analysis: per ½-cup serving
CALORIES: 231   PROTEIN: 3 grams   CARBS.: 42 grams   TOTAL FAT: 6 grams   SAT. FAT: 1 gram
POLY. FAT: 1 gram   MONO. FAT: 4 grams   CHOLES.: 0 mg   FIBER: 3 grams (Sol. 2 grams)
SODIUM: 24 mgs

Roasted Sweet Potatoes with Rosemary

Rosemary enhances the natural sweetness of the potatoes to produce crispy and delectable roasted potatoes.

Yield: 4 cups; 6 (⅔-cup) servings
Preparation time: 35 minutes

1½ pounds sweet potatoes
1½ tablespoons olive oil
2 teaspoons minced fresh rosemary
½ teaspoon salt
¼ teaspoon pepper

Lightly coat a 15 x 10-inch baking sheet with olive oil spray. Position a rack in lower third of oven. Preheat oven to 425 degrees Fahrenheit.

Scrub sweet potatoes well. Rinse and dry completely. Cut sweet potatoes into ¾-inch dice.

Place sweet potatoes on prepared baking sheet and drizzle with olive oil. Sprinkle with rosemary, salt, and pepper. Toss well to coat and place baking sheet on lower rack. Bake about 30 minutes, or until golden outside and tender inside. Turn potatoes once during baking.

Rosemary Factoid: Rosemary contains a phytochemical called *carvacrol,* which has shown significant antifungal and antibacterial activity. It has been studied specifically for its ability to interfere with candidiasis growth.

Nutrient Analysis: per ⅔-cup serving
Calories: 102   Protein: 1 gram   Carbs.: 16 grams   Total fat: 4 grams   Sat. fat: 0.5 gram
Poly. fat: 0 gram   Mono. fat: 3 grams   Choles.: 0 mg   Fiber: 2 grams (Sol. 1 gram)
Sodium: 203 mgs

Red Pepper Confit

There's no mistake in the yield: Four bell peppers simmer and melt into an intense reduction. This buttery confit is the ultimate essence of bell peppery flavor. It stands up well to grilled foods and makes an inventive condiment for a sandwich or bruschetta.

YIELD: 1 CUP; 8 (2-TABLESPOON) SERVINGS
PREPARATION TIME: 45 MINUTES

2 tablespoons olive oil
4 large red bell peppers (about 1 pound), cut into julienne strips
¼ cup sorghum syrup
1 cup dry red wine
2 tablespoons balsamic vinegar

Heat oil in a large sauté pan over medium heat. Add bell peppers and sorghum syrup. Cover and cook over low heat, 25 minutes, stirring occasionally. Watch carefully to avoid burning. Mixture will be nearly dry when finished.

Add wine and vinegar. Return to a boil and simmer, uncovered, until juices have thickened, about 15 minutes. Serve warm or at room temperature.

Bell Pepper Factoid: Ounce for ounce, red bell peppers have twice the vitamin C content of green bell peppers or oranges.

Nutrient Analysis: per 2-tablespoon serving

CALORIES: 107   PROTEIN: 1 gram   CARBS.: 14 grams   TOTAL FAT: 3 grams   SAT. FAT: 0 gram
POLY. FAT: 0 gram   MONO. FAT: 3 grams   CHOLES.: 0 mg   FIBER: 2 grams   SODIUM: 5 mgs

Pumpkin Butter

If you're a pumpkin pie fan, you'll love this creamy spread. Try it on muffins or whole-grain toast, or stir a spoonful into your hot cereal.

YIELD: 4½ CUPS; 6 (¼-CUP) SERVINGS
PREPARATION TIME: 40 MINUTES

> *3⅓ cups pumpkin purée (29 ounces)*
> *1½ cups unflavored soymilk*
> *¾ cup sorghum syrup*
> *2 teaspoons ground ginger*
> *1 teaspoon ground cinnamon*
> *½ teaspoon ground cloves*
> *½ teaspoon ground nutmeg*
> *¼ teaspoon ground cardamom*
> *Pinch salt*

Combine pumpkin, soymilk, sorghum syrup, and spices in a deep 3-quart saucepan; stir well. Bring mixture just to a boil over medium heat. Immediately reduce heat, cover slightly, and simmer until thickened, about 30 minutes, stirring frequently. Caution: As the mixture thickens, it tends to spatter and may burn skin.

Pour into clean, sterilized jars and seal. Cool and store in the refrigerator for up to 1 month.

Pumpkin Factoid: The bright color of pumpkin roars that it's loaded with a powerful antioxidant—beta-carotene. Beta-carotene is a plant carotenoid that converts to vitamin A in the body.

Nutrient Analysis: per ¼-cup serving

CALORIES: 59 PROTEIN: 1 gram CARBS.: 3 grams TOTAL FAT: 0.5 gram SAT. FAT: 0 gram
POLY. FAT: 0 gram MONO. FAT: 0 gram CHOLES.: 0 mg FIBER: 1 gram SODIUM: 4 mgs

Sweet Mango Lassi

Lassi (or *lhassi*) is an Indian yogurt drink. A savory lassi may be flavored with spices such as cumin and may even contain salt. This sweet frothy lassi is enriched with creamy mango. It's typical of the sweet lassis often served to balance the heat of spicy curry dishes.

YIELD: 2½ CUPS; 2 (1¼-CUP) SERVINGS
PREPARATION TIME: 5 MINUTES

> ½ cup plain soy yogurt (*see Note below*)
> 1 cup vanilla soymilk
> 6 ice cubes
> ½ cup chopped mango
> 2 teaspoons sorghum syrup or dark honey
> ½ teaspoon grated lemon peel
> ½ teaspoon pure vanilla extract

Combine all the ingredients in a blender or food processor and blend until the ice has been crushed and the liquid is frothy. Pour into glasses and serve immediately.

NOTE: Soy yogurt is slightly sweeter than its dairy counterpart. Soy yogurt can be found in health food stores and some supermarkets.

Mango Factoid: The content of carotenoid antioxidants present in the pulp of the mango increases with ripeness.

Nutrient Analysis: per 1¼-cup serving

CALORIES: 137   PROTEIN: 5 grams   CARBS.: 22 grams   TOTAL FAT: 3 grams   SAT. FAT: 1 gram

POLY. FAT: 1 gram   MONO. FAT: 1 gram   CHOLES.: 0 gram   FIBER: 2 grams (Sol. 1 gram)

SODIUM: 23 mgs

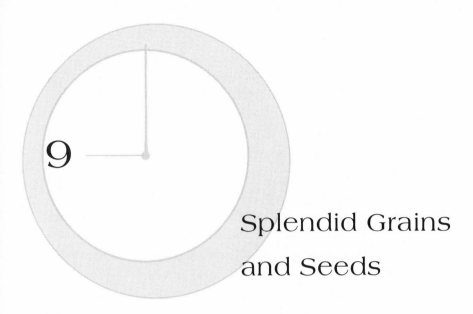

9

Splendid Grains and Seeds

Whole grains rocked the cradle of civilization. They have sustained families and continents as food *and* as treasure. Gingery rice porridge in Beijing, soft corn tortillas in Lima, nutty kasha in Moscow—grains are a familiar and comforting constant, our global common thread.

But whole grains have fallen from favor recently. Too much work, too time consuming, and too unfamiliar now that we have so many choices that are tasty, fast, and economical. But "fast" is a dead giveaway for a grain that is refined. And though refining pares back preparation time, it also peels away the most valuable parts of a whole grain.

There are plenty of reasons to love grains au naturel. Whole grains are versatile, inexpensive, surprisingly easy to prepare, and *amazingly* flavorful. The grain family includes barley, corn, millet, oats, rice, rye, sorghum, and wheat—all great sources of protein, B vitamins, and fiber. But if you thought that fiber is the only thing that grains have going for them, you've missed the boat. Whole grains are "hot," and they're *teeming* with anti-aging phytochemicals.

True, grains lack the vibrant colors that proclaim the phytochemical bounty of many fruits and vegetables. Berries, citrus, and grapes are the pipeline to polyphenols. Yellow- and red-hued fruits and vegetables are the gateway to carotenoids. And phytosterols, the cholesterol clones, are found in avocados, soy, nuts, and seeds. But whole grains have all three groups of phytochemicals. This translates to antiaging (antioxidant) activity on par with many fruits and *exceeding* most vegetables.

Whole grains are similar in structure. Bran is the outer layer of a grain kernel. The seed is the germ. And the largest part is the endosperm, which is all that remains after refining. It still contains protein and carbohydrate, but the precious fiber and phytochemical cargo are sacrificed in refining. Valuable micronutrients such as folic acid, magnesium, and vitamin E are lost, too.

Creatures of habit, we timidly sample only a smattering of Mother Earth's offerings, but an occasional bowl of oats or a slice of whole-grain bread just won't do it. If you're seeking the Holy Grail for antiaging foods, take another look at your options.

OATS

The reputed "breakfast grain," oats are extraordinary in their nutrient abundance. Unlike many grains, unrefined oats are the rule, not the exception. Keeping the grain intact preserves its antiaging assets, since many reside in the outer or bran layer, which is the first to go in refining. Oats possess lignans, a plant form of estrogen that helps maintain bone strength. In addition, the unique nutritional profile of oats, which includes avenanthramides (polyphenols), saponins, and several types of fiber, promotes oxidative balance and heart health.

The abundance of beta-glucan fiber in oats has incredible healing powers. Like other soluble fibers, it binds cholesterol in the intestinal tract, thus contributing to lowered LDL (bad cholesterol). Because it is an insoluble fiber, it also moderates the release of glucose into the bloodstream, improving blood sugar control. One of the functions unique to oat fiber is its effect on promoting blood pressure control.

Add spark to your breakfast and stoke your antiaging fire with chewy, nutty Stop the Clock! Grainola or Muesli and Dried Fruit.

WHEAT

Wheat is considered the "bread grain" because it contains gluten-forming proteins that give structure to baked goods. Wheat flour is the result of grinding wheat kernels, or "berries." The kernel consists of three components: bran, which is the outer covering of the kernel; the germ, which is the innermost part of the kernel; and the endosperm, the part of the kernel that makes white flour. During milling, the three parts are separated and re-combined according to the type of flour desired. Whole-wheat or stone-ground flour re-sults from either grinding the whole-wheat kernel or recombining the endosperm, germ, and bran that have been separated during milling.

Though refined wheat flour comprises countless "empty-calorie" foods, its unrefined counterparts are loaded with antiaging ammo. Bulgur is made from whole-wheat berries that are steamed, partially de-branned, dried, and crushed or cracked. A meal with bulgur also provides protein and fiber. The result is steady energy that lasts long beyond mealtime. Fiber also promotes regularity, increases satiety, and thus may help keep obesity at bay.

Available in coarse, medium, and fine grinds, bulgur is a staple in the Middle Eastern diet. Usually seen on the lunch or dinner table, it's an ideal breakfast grain. Climb out of your morning rut and indulge in the exotic flavors of *Kutia* (Lemony Poppy Seed Porridge) or Casbah Bulgur.

CORN

A warm wedge of nutty cornbread is a fixture on the Southern table. Although it differs in color from the brown and beige grains, corn has many of the same nutrients. A rich reserve of insoluble fiber, whole-grain corn provides bulk and speeds the passage of food through-out the digestive tract, promoting regularity and potentially reducing the risk of colon can-cer. A relative of beta-carotene, xeaxanthin is an antiaging phytochemical that gives corn its amber complexion. Xeaxanthin has been studied for its role in enhancing immune function and in fighting cancer and macular degeneration. Corn also has proteins called *protease in-hibitors* that appear to suppress initiation and promotion of cancer growth.

This golden grain gives comfort food a new meaning when you consider its antiaging benefits. Satisfy your soul with a mound of Creamy Stone-Ground Polenta or a bowl of warm Indian Pudding.

SORGHUM

One of the most astonishing grains has managed to keep a low profile despite the fact that its antioxidant powers are unrivaled. Haven't heard of sorghum? You will. This amazing grain is about to stand the world on its ear with its antiaging powers. Sorghum has been around for eons, and in some parts of the world it is the principal food. Americans lag way behind in consumption, but the tide is about to turn.

Distinct from the sorghum syrup plant, sorghum grain has an incredible antioxidant bounty, particularly in its bran layer. The antioxidants include plant forms of vitamin E (tocopherols and tocotrienols), phytins, anthocyanins, phenols, and tannins, which collectively inhibit the ravaging effects of free radicals that can lead to cataracts, cancer, arthritis, brain dysfunction, and heart disease. And, compared with that of wheat, sorghum's bran layer has 45 percent more insoluble fiber. Turn on the oven and bake a batch of protection with Whole-Wheat Pita Bread.

MILLET

Millet is as old as the hills. This biblical grain is loaded with B vitamins, potassium, and a slew of phytochemicals, including sterols, phytases, lignans, ellagic acid, isoprenoids, and saponins. This powerful posse has the means to fight cancer and heart disease by a variety of methods.

BUCKWHEAT

Despite its name, buckwheat, a grainlike seed, isn't a wheat at all. Porous and absorbent, it's quick and easy to prepare. Kasha is the result of toasting buckwheat. This process separates the grains and adds a nutty flavor. Buckwheat contains an antioxidant called *rutin,* which is thought to strengthen capillaries (tiny blood vessels) and may be beneficial in controlling blood pressure. It is also rich in fiber, protein, B vitamins, calcium, iron, phosphorus, and potassium. Savor the nutty grains of millet and toasted buckwheat in Mahogany Millet with Kasha, Dried Blueberries, Mango, and Toasted Walnuts.

SEEDS

Don't let the size of a seed beguile you. Its meager measure harbors a titanic arsenal of anti-aging weapons. Sesame, sunflower, and pumpkin seeds are all rich sources of protein, fiber, and phytosterols, the cholesterol clones. Pumpkin seeds are particularly rich in beta-sitosterol, a sterol thought to suppress the conversion of testosterone to dihydrotestosterone, a harmful form of the hormone, particularly to men over forty who are at risk for a condition called *benign prostatic hyperplasia* (BPH), enlargement of the prostate gland. Pumpkin seeds are thought to suppress the hormonal conversion, thus reducing the risk for BPH.

Pumpkin seeds are also rich in an amino acid called *lysine*. Researchers hope to discover a decrease in cold sore infections with lysine use. Turn back your clock and set your mouth in motion with the exotic flavor medley of Chicken Mole with Pumpkin and Sesame Seeds or Cara's Ginger Crackers.

Open sesame. Unlock the treasure of this tiny nutty seed and you'll find a frenzy of antiaging activity. No wonder sesame keeps a place in pantries around the world. Toasted seeds, creamy tahini paste, and aromatic oil are celebrated forms. In addition to protein, sterols, and fiber, sesame seeds are a stellar source of calcium and heart-healthy fats. They also contain several forms of vitamin E, which are believed to play a role in the prevention of aging-related diseases such as heart disease and cancer. Feast on sesame's treasures and let its seasoning awaken in creamy Tangy Mustard-Tahini Sauce.

Chicken Mole with Pumpkin and Sesame Seeds

*M*ole (pronounced MOH-lay) is a magical sauce with a complex blend of spices. Most Mexican families have their own prized combination. Typically, mole is made with a fragrant blend of spices and a surprising ingredient, cocoa powder. Smoky and rich, there is a subtle undertone of chocolate, which is redefined in this riot of flavors. Serve with Creamy Stone-Ground Polenta (page 151) or brown rice.

YIELD: 1½ QUARTS; 6 (1-CUP) SERVINGS

PREPARATION TIME: 1 HOUR

1½ medium red onions, cut into eighths

2 torn or crumbled corn tortillas

⅓ cup pitted, slivered dried plums

½ cup dry red wine

¼ cup toasted almonds (see Note, page 133)

2 tablespoons pumpkin seeds

2 tablespoons toasted sesame seeds (see Note, page 98)

1 teaspoon coriander seeds

¼ teaspoon anise seeds

2 chipotle chiles or 2 dried chipotle chiles reconstituted in 2 tablespoons
    warm water (see Note, page 63)

1 teaspoon ground cinnamon

¼ teaspoon ground cloves

2 tablespoons unsweetened natural cocoa powder

2 tablespoons olive oil

1 pound boneless, skinless chicken breasts, cut into bite-size pieces

1 cup peeled, halved, seeded, chopped tomatoes (see Note, page 195)

½ cup finely diced green bell pepper

1 cup tomato sauce

2 tablespoons minced garlic
2 cups fat-free, low-sodium chicken broth
Salt and pepper to taste

Garnish:
2 tablespoons fresh chopped cilantro, without stems

Combine onions, tortillas, plums, wine, almonds, seeds, chiles, spices, cocoa powder, and 1 tablespoon of the olive oil in the bowl of a food processor; process to a smooth paste.

Heat remaining 1 tablespoon oil in a Dutch oven or 4-quart pan over medium-high heat. Brown chicken pieces on both sides and remove from pan.

Add spice paste to same pan over medium heat. If paste is very thick, add ¼ cup water. Cook paste until bubbly and fragrant, about 5 minutes, stirring frequently. Add tomatoes, bell pepper, tomato sauce, garlic, and 1¼ cups broth to pan. Bring to a boil. Reduce heat to low, cover, and simmer for 10 minutes. Add enough of remaining broth to achieve a smooth sauce with the consistency of thick cream.

Return chicken to pan, cover, and simmer until chicken is just cooked through and vegetables are tender, about 5 minutes.

Season with salt and pepper. Garnish with cilantro.

Pumpkin Factoid: Pumpkin seeds are at least 50 percent oil by weight. For the most part, the oil is composed of healthy, unsaturated fatty acids. The seeds are also a great source of the antioxidant vitamin E.

Nutrient Analysis: per 1-cup serving

CALORIES: 296   PROTEIN: 25 grams   CARBS.: 24 grams   TOTAL FAT: 11 grams   SAT. FAT: 2 grams

POLY. FAT: 3 grams   MONO. FAT: 6 grams   CHOLES.: 44 mgs   FIBER: 5 grams (Sol. 1 gram)

SODIUM: 133 mgs

Casbah Bulgur

Bulgur is a staple in North Africa and is made from wheat. This dish combines the ingredients of a traditional couscous, but the cooking method has been simplified to save time and minimize fat. Coarse bulgur also has more nutrients and fiber than refined couscous. The combination of whole grains, vegetables, raisins, and spices gives it an intriguing blend of textures and flavors.

YIELD: 4 CUPS; 6 (¾-CUP) SERVINGS
PREPARATION TIME: 25 MINUTES

> 2 tablespoons olive oil
> 1 cup coarsely ground bulgur
> 1 teaspoon ground cinnamon
> ¾ teaspoon ground turmeric
> 2 cups fat-free chicken or vegetable broth
> ½ cup finely chopped yellow onion
> ½ cup finely diced red bell pepper
> ½ cup finely diced yellow bell pepper
> 1 teaspoon minced garlic
> 2 teaspoons chopped Preserved Lemon peel (page 48)
>   or grated lemon peel
> ½ cup cooked garbanzo beans
> ½ cup raisins
> Salt and pepper to taste

Garnish:
2 tablespoons chopped fresh cilantro, without stems

Heat 1 tablespoon of the oil in a 2-quart saucepan over medium heat. Pour in bulgur and spices. Cook, stirring, until spices are fragrant and bulgur begins to toast, about 3 minutes. Carefully pour in broth. Stir and bring to a boil. Reduce heat to low, cover, and simmer 5 minutes. Turn off heat.

Meanwhile, heat the remaining 1 tablespoon oil in a large sauté pan over medium-high heat. Add onion and bell peppers and sauté until softened. Add garlic and cook for 1 minute; do not brown garlic.

Add lemon peel, beans, raisins, and sautéed vegetables to the cooked bulgur and stir to combine. Season with salt and pepper. Garnish with cilantro. Serve hot.

Bulgur Factoid: Bulgur is an ancient food whose use dates back to biblical times. The whole-wheat kernel is soaked, precooked, dried, and then cracked. The result is quicker cooking.

Nutrient Analysis: per ¾-cup serving

CALORIES: 204 PROTEIN: 7 grams CARBS.: 35 grams TOTAL FAT: 5 grams SAT. FAT: 1 gram

POLY. FAT: 1 gram MONO. FAT: 3 grams CHOLES.: 0 mg FIBER: 7 grams (Sol. 1 gram)

SODIUM: 64 mgs

Creamy Stone-Ground Polenta

This soft polenta is an easy whole-grain alternative to pasta or potatoes. Add your favorite herbs or spices to create family favorites. Serve the polenta with fresh tomato sauce or spicy Mexican food.

YIELD: 3½ CUPS; 7 (½-CUP) SERVINGS

PREPARATION TIME: 30 MINUTES

> *5 cups water*
> *1 tablespoon olive oil*
> *1 teaspoon salt*
> *1½ cups stone-ground cornmeal*

Bring water, olive oil, and salt to a boil in a heavy 3-quart saucepan over medium heat. Whisk in cornmeal in a slow stream. Reduce heat to low, cover, and cook, stirring frequently, until polenta is thick and creamy, about 20 minutes.

> *Corn Factoid:* Corn contains protease inhibitors, which suppress cancer growth during the initiation and promotion stages. It also contains phytosterols and phytostanols, that inhibit the absorption of cholesterol from the small intestine.

Nutrient Analysis: per ½-cup serving

CALORIES: 111   PROTEIN: 2 grams   CARBS.: 20 grams   TOTAL FAT: 3 grams   SAT. FAT: 0 gram
POLY. FAT: 0 gram   MONO. FAT: 2 grams   CHOLES.: 3 mgs   FIBER: 4 grams   SODIUM: 344 mgs

Mahogany Millet with Kasha, Dried Blueberries, Mango, and Toasted Walnuts

This rustic cereal is a vision of autumn. Lacquered grains of chewy millet are flecked with sweet dried blueberries and mango. Pan-toasting the millet before cooking gives it a wonderful flavor and a nutty crunch. For a softer porridgelike consistency, add an extra ¼ cup of soymilk during cooking. Serve with additional soymilk and fruit if desired.

YIELD: 1 QUART; 8 (½-CUP) SERVINGS
PREPARATION TIME: 40 MINUTES

1 tablespoon olive oil
¾ cup millet
¼ cup kasha
2¼ cups vanilla soymilk
¼ cup sorghum syrup
½ teaspoon ground cardamom

½ cup dried blueberries
¼ cup finely diced dried mango
½ cup chopped toasted walnuts (see Note, page 31)

Heat oil in a 2-quart saucepan over medium heat. Add millet and cook, stirring occasionally, until lightly toasted, about 3 minutes. Add kasha, soymilk, sorghum syrup, and cardamom. Bring mixture to a boil. Cover, reduce heat to low, and simmer until most of the liquid has been absorbed but mixture is still loose, about 25 minutes.

Remove from heat and stir in blueberries, mango, and walnuts.

Buckwheat Factoid: Untoasted buckwheat or groats are as versatile as rice. For a yield of 2½ cups cooked groats, add 1 cup dry groats to 2 cups water or broth and cook for about 20 minutes.

Millet Factoid: Millet contains phytic acid and phytate. Phytic acid lowers cholesterol, and phytate reduces the risk of cancer.

Nutrient Analysis: per ½-cup serving

CALORIES: 255   PROTEIN: 6 grams   CARBS.: 41 grams   TOTAL FAT: 8 grams   SAT. FAT: 1 gram
POLY. FAT: 3 grams   MONO. FAT: 4 grams   CHOLES.: 0 mg   FIBER: 4 grams   SODIUM: 35 mgs

Whole-Wheat Pita Bread

"You make your own pita bread? There are many terrific whole-grain pita breads on the market today. Why bother?" I can hear my sister now. I couldn't resist the temptation to spike my dough with antioxidant-rich sorghum flour and a hint of sorghum syrup. Yes, it takes extra time, but the result is well worth the effort.

YIELD: 20 (6-INCH) PITA BREADS
PREPARATION TIME: 2 HOURS

2 packages active dry yeast
3½ cups unbleached all-purpose flour
2 cups unflavored soymilk
2 tablespoons sorghum syrup or dark honey
3 tablespoons olive oil
1½ cups whole-wheat flour
½ cup sorghum flour
1 teaspoon salt
Cornmeal for dusting baking sheets

Combine yeast and 2 cups of the unbleached all-purpose flour in a large mixing bowl. Warm the soymilk, sorghum syrup, and olive oil in a 1-quart saucepan to 120 degrees Fahrenheit. Add the milk mixture to the yeast and flour mixture; beat 30 seconds with an electric mixer. Scrape sides of bowl. Beat 3 minutes at high speed.

Let dough rest 10 minutes to allow the yeast to activate and bubble.

Mix in whole-wheat flour, sorghum flour, salt, and 1 cup of the remaining all-purpose flour to make a moderately stiff dough. Add an additional ½ cup all-purpose flour if needed to make a smooth dough. Turn out on a floured surface and knead until smooth and elastic.

Place dough in a large mixing bowl that has been sprayed with olive oil cooking spray; turn over to coat both sides of dough. Cover and let rise in a warm place until doubled, about 45 minutes.

Punch down the dough; cover and let it rest for 10 minutes. Transfer dough to a clean, floured surface. Divide dough into about 20 equal pieces, each about ¼ cup of dough. Roll each piece into a ball about 2 inches in diameter. Using a rolling pin, flatten each ball into a 6-inch circle. Use extra flour as needed to prevent sticking. Cover the circles with a clean towel and let them rest for about 30 minutes.

Preheat oven to 450 degrees Fahrenheit. Dust ungreased baking sheets with cornmeal. A 15 x 10-inch baking sheet will hold about 5 circles without touching.

Bake about 7 minutes, or until puffed and very lightly browned on the bottom. If bread is allowed to brown during baking, it will not be soft enough to allow for stuffing the pita bread. Remove from the oven. Immediately cover the bread with a clean towel. Cool completely and wrap the bread airtight.

Sorghum Flour Factoid: Sorghum flour is the predominant source of nutrition in some parts of the world. It is gluten free and very high in antioxidants. It doesn't have all the attributes of wheat flour, so it can't be substituted equally, but it's a great way to "infuse" your favorite recipes with an antioxidant boost.

Nutrient Analysis: per 6-inch pita bread

CALORIES: 143 PROTEIN: 4 grams CARBS.: 25 grams TOTAL FAT: 3 grams SAT. FAT: 0 gram POLY. FAT: 0 gram MONO. FAT: 2 grams CHOLES.: 0 mg FIBER: 2 grams SODIUM: 121 mgs

Bengali Breakfast Grains

A whisper of exotic spices results in complex flavors and a stunningly simple breakfast treat.

YIELD: 3 CUPS; 6 (½-CUP) SERVINGS
PREPARATION TIME: 25 MINUTES

1 tablespoon olive oil
1 cup coarsely ground bulgur
1½ teaspoons fennel seeds
2 cups vanilla soymilk or 2 cups unflavored soymilk plus 1 teaspoon
*   pure vanilla extract*
½ teaspoon ground cardamom
½ teaspoon ground cinnamon
Pinch nutmeg

Garnish:
½ cup dried blueberries (about 3 ounces) or other dried or fresh berries

Heat oil in a 2-quart saucepan over medium heat. Add bulgur and fennel seeds and cook, stirring frequently, until bulgur is light golden brown, about 5 minutes.

Remove saucepan from heat. Carefully stir in soymilk and spices. Return to heat and bring to a boil. Reduce heat to low, cover, and simmer until most, but not all, of the liquid has been absorbed, about 12 minutes.

Spoon into serving dishes. Garnish with blueberries and serve.

Bulgur Factoid: Bulgur is made by boiling whole-wheat berries, then roasting and grinding them to the desired texture. Because it is precooked, bulgur is relatively quick to prepare.

Nutrient Analysis: per ½-cup serving

CALORIES: 210   PROTEIN: 6 grams   CARBS.: 39 grams   TOTAL FAT: 4 grams   SAT. FAT: 1 gram

POLY. FAT: 1 gram   MONO. FAT: 1 gram   CHOLES.: 0 mg   FIBER: 6 grams (Sol. 1 gram)

SODIUM: 51 mgs

Stop the Clock! Grainola

The ingredients for this addictive recipe can be combined in minutes. Slowly toasting the grainola in a low oven allows for even browning. This large recipe yields 4 quarts of grainola, but it won't last long. Store it in the freezer for optimal freshness. Serve with milk and additional fresh or dried fruit if desired.

YIELD: 16 CUPS (3½ POUNDS); 32 (½-CUP) SERVINGS
PREPARATION TIME: 1 HOUR

6 cups old-fashioned rolled oats
1 cup low-fat soy flour
1 cup raw wheat germ (see Note, page 158)
1 cup nonfat dry milk powder
1 cup wheat or oat bran
½ cup shredded unsweetened coconut (optional)
½ cup chopped walnuts
½ cup raw sunflower seeds (see Note, page 158)
⅓ cup untoasted sesame seeds (see Note, page 158)
¾ cup olive oil
1 cup sorghum syrup or dark honey
3 tablespoons pure vanilla extract
1 cup raisins or dried berries

Preheat oven to 250 degrees Fahrenheit. Combine oats, soy flour, wheat germ, dry milk, bran, coconut (if using), walnuts, and seeds in a large mixing bowl.

Combine oil and sorghum syrup in a 1-quart saucepan over medium heat. Heat until mixture is warm and well combined. Do not boil. Remove from heat and stir in vanilla.

Pour oil mixture over dry ingredients and combine well. Divide mixture between 2 ungreased 15 x 10-inch baking sheets and spread evenly. Bake 1 hour, stirring every 20 minutes to ensure even browning. Stir in raisins or berries during last 10 minutes of baking. Cool completely and store in airtight containers.

NOTE: It is important that the wheat germ, sunflower seeds, and sesame seeds are raw and not toasted; otherwise they will burn during the slow toasting process. These items are available in health food stores.

Sunflower Seed Factoid: Sunflower seeds contain selenium, vitamin E, and phenolic acid—a wallop of antiaging nutrition.

Nutrient Analysis: per ½-cup serving

CALORIES: 213   PROTEIN: 7 grams   CARBS.: 27 grams   TOTAL FAT: 9 grams   SAT. FAT: 1 gram
POLY. FAT: 3 grams   MONO. FAT: 5 grams   CHOLES.: 0 mg   FIBER: 4 grams (Sol. 1 gram)
SODIUM: 17 mgs

Variation

Muesli and Dried Fruit

½ cup Stop the Clock! Grainola (see page 157)
½ cup unflavored soymilk
¼ cup dried blueberries or other dried berry

Combine Grainola, soymilk, and blueberries in a serving bowl or storage container. Cover and refrigerate several hours or overnight.

Before serving, top with additional fresh fruit if desired.

Tangy Mustard-Tahini Sauce

This tangy sauce is an addictive condiment. Try it with Falafel Sandwiches (page 177), Chicken Shwarma (page 78), or your own favorite sandwich. It will keep for several weeks in the refrigerator, if it lasts that long.

YIELD: 2 CUPS; 32 (1-TABLESPOON) SERVINGS
PREPARATION TIME: 5 MINUTES

⅔ cup Dijon mustard
½ cup tahini (see Note, page below)
½ cup soft silken tofu
⅓ cup fresh lime juice

Combine all ingredients in a blender and blend until smooth. For a thinner sauce, add 1 to 2 tablespoons water. Pour into an airtight container and refrigerate.

Tahini Factoid: Aside from being eaten whole, sesame seeds are commonly ground into pastes. Those with thicker texture are referred to as sesame butter, and thinner pastes are called tahini.

Nutrient Analysis: per 1-tablespoon serving

CALORIES: 32   PROTEIN: 1 gram   CARBS.: 2 grams   TOTAL FAT: 3 grams   SAT. FAT: 0 gram
POLY. FAT: 1 gram   MONO. FAT: 1 gram   CHOLES.: 0 mg   FIBER: 0 gram   SODIUM: 128 mgs

Indian Pudding

Indian pudding was a popular dessert in the American colonies in the 1700s. The colonists' recipe was similar to a Native American dish called *supawn*. A contemporary twist on a very old-fashioned favorite, this homespun pudding is great for breakfast, too.

YIELD: 5 CUPS; 10 (½-CUP) SERVINGS
PREPARATION TIME: 45 MINUTES

¾ cup stone-ground cornmeal
½ teaspoon salt
2 teaspoons ground cinnamon
2 teaspoons ground ginger
4 cups unflavored soymilk
¾ cup sorghum syrup

Preheat oven to 350 degrees Fahrenheit. Lightly coat a 1½-quart baking or soufflé dish with olive oil cooking spray.

Combine dry ingredients in a small mixing bowl and set aside.

Combine soymilk and sorghum syrup in a 3-quart saucepan. Heat over medium-high heat to just about boiling, stirring often. Slowly whisk in dry ingredients. Cook, whisking constantly, until mixture comes to a full boil, about 1 minute. Reduce heat to low and simmer until mixture just begins to thicken, about 5 minutes, whisking frequently.

Remove cornmeal mixture from heat and pour into prepared baking dish. Bake, uncovered, about 20 minutes. Stir pudding and bake another 20 minutes. Remove from oven and allow to cool slightly. Serve warm.

Stone-ground Cornmeal Factoid: Stone-ground cornmeal is available in most health food stores. Because the germ has not been removed, its nutrient is quite superior to ordinary cornmeal. The preservation of the germ increases the fat content, thus decreasing the shelf life. It should be refrigerated.

Nutrient Analysis: per ½-cup serving

CALORIES: 142   PROTEIN: 4 grams   CARBS.: 27 grams   TOTAL FAT: 2 grams   SAT. FAT: 0 gram

POLY. FAT: 1 gram   MONO. FAT: 0 gram   CHOLES.: 0 mg   FIBER: 2 grams (Sol. 1 gram)

SODIUM: 47 mgs

Variation

Pour ¼ cup toasted walnuts (see Note, page 31) and ¼ cup dried berries (blueberries, cranberries, or cherries) into the pudding dish after the first 20 minutes of baking. Stir well and then continue baking as directed for 20 minutes longer.

Cara's Ginger Crackers

Created the day of her wedding, these eponymous treats are crackly crisp and simply addictive. With a hint of sweetness, they are a perfect snack, plain or slathered with jam. Savor them with a steaming cup of tea or your favorite glass of red wine or Port.

YIELD: 24 CRACKERS

PREPARATION TIME: 1 HOUR

¾ cup unbleached all-purpose flour
¼ cup sorghum flour
½ cup raw wheat germ
½ cup oat or wheat bran
1 teaspoon ground ginger
1 teaspoon mustard powder
1 teaspoon baking powder
½ teaspoon salt
¼ cup olive oil
¼ cup sorghum syrup

1 large egg white

½ teaspoon pure vanilla extract

2 tablespoons ground flaxseed (see Note, page 000)

2 tablespoons sesame seeds

2 tablespoons poppy seeds

About 1 tablespoon unflavored soymilk or water

Combine dry ingredients in a small mixing bowl.

Combine oil, sorghum syrup, egg white, and vanilla in a medium mixing bowl. Add dry ingredients; mix well. Stir in flaxseed, sesame seeds, and poppy seeds, and 1 tablespoon soymilk just until combined. If necessary, add enough soymilk to make the dough hold together.

Place a 12-inch piece of aluminum foil on a flat work surface. Place a 12-inch piece of plastic wrap directly on top of foil. Form a 6-inch-long by 2-inch-diameter cylinder of dough 2 inches from one long edge of the plastic wrap. Roll up the dough to make a tightly sealed cylinder. Twist each end to compact and remove air bubbles. You will have a solid symmetrical roll. Place in freezer for 2 hours or until very firm.

To bake the crackers, preheat oven to 350 degrees Fahrenheit. Remove dough from freezer and unwrap. Working quickly, slice the dough into ¼-inch-thick rounds with a sharp thin knife and place directly on an ungreased baking sheet.

Bake about 12 minutes, or until lightly browned. Let cool 5 minutes on baking sheet before removing with a metal spatula.

Flaxseed Factoid: Flaxseeds add nutty flavor when sprinkled on cereal, soups, or salads. Flaxseed and flax oil contain unsaturated fats so they spoil quickly; store them in the refrigerator. Flaxseed can be used to replace fat in some recipes, because of the high oil content.

Nutrient Analysis: per cracker

CALORIES: 76 PROTEIN: 2 grams CARBS.: 10 grams TOTAL FAT: 4 grams SAT. FAT: 1 gram

POLY. FAT: 1 gram MONO. FAT: 2 grams CHOLES.: 0 mg FIBER: 1 gram SODIUM: 73 mgs

Kutia (Lemony Poppy Seed Porridge)

Kutia is a sacred ritual dish of the Ukraine and a classic holiday meal. This crunchy sweet grain dish is usually the first of a traditional twelve-course feast served just after sundown on Christmas Eve. Though usually served cold, it is delicious warm for breakfast.

YIELD: 2 QUARTS; 12 (¾-CUP) SERVINGS
PREPARATION TIME: 45 MINUTES

1 tablespoon olive oil
2 cups coarsely ground bulgur
4½ cups vanilla soymilk
Pinch salt
½ cup chopped, toasted walnuts, almonds, or pecans (see Note, page 31)
1 cup chopped dried cranberries, cherries, or raisins
2 tablespoons sorghum syrup or dark honey
1 teaspoon pure vanilla extract
¼ cup poppy seeds
2 teaspoons grated citrus peel (lemon, orange, or tangerine)

Heat olive oil in a 2-quart saucepan over medium heat. Add bulgur and cook until evenly toasted, about 4 minutes, stirring constantly. Carefully stir in soymilk and salt; heat until hot but do not boil. Reduce heat to low, cover, and simmer until creamy but loose, about 13 minutes. Remove from heat.

Add nuts, cranberries, sorghum syrup, vanilla, poppy seeds, and citrus peel; stir to combine. *Kutia* may be served warm or chilled.

Poppy Seed Factoid: Not all poppy seeds are gray. Pale golden seeds are common in India; brown seeds prevail in Turkey; and European poppy seeds are blue-gray.

Nutrient Analysis: per ¾-cup serving

CALORIES: 208   PROTEIN: 7 grams   CARBS.: 31 grams   TOTAL FAT: 8 grams   SAT. FAT: 1 gram

POLY. FAT: 2 grams   MONO. FAT: 3 grams   CHOLES.: 0 mg   FIBER: 7 grams (Sol. 1 gram)

SODIUM: 16 mgs

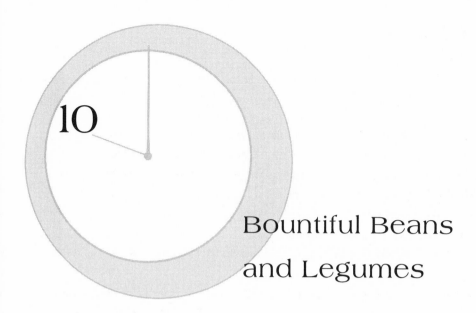

10

Bountiful Beans and Legumes

Four centuries ago, a respected holistic physician named Nicholas Culpeper prescribed citrus juices to strengthen the heart and nutmeg to ease pain in the joints. He also advocated fava bean juice to remove spots and wrinkles from the skin, and the legume became legendary. Antiaging foods are not new, but Dr. C was ahead of his time.

Legumes are a culinary paradox. The least expensive group of foods, they have priceless antiaging benefits. Hundreds of beans, peas, peanuts, and lentils belong to the legume family, offering a legion of benefits as diverse as their varieties. Edible seeds that grow in pods, legumes are an excellent source of fiber. They're also rich in folic acid, calcium, iron, potassium, zinc, and antioxidants. And their high protein and complex carbohydrate profile provides steady energy that lasts well beyond mealtimes.

Cooks around the world dish up familiar and comforting legume meals to start each day—from Mexican refried beans to Japanese miso soup. Many of their menus are built on a base of versatile legumes.

FAVA BEANS

Ancient Romans had so much respect for delectable legumes that their nobility derived their family names from them. The Fabius family moniker is a testament to reverence for the fava bean. And in France, the fava, also known as the broad bean, is celebrated for an entire season. In the Middle Eastern diet, fresh, dried, and canned fava beans are a mainstay of everyday fare. A native dish, *foul muddamas* or *foul,* is a fava bean stew that's a standard at mealtime—from breakfast through dinner. Fava beans don't have mass appeal in the United States—yet. But once the antiaging buzz is out on this legume, fava beans will attract new fans.

One of the bean family's prized claims is its unbeatable amount of soluble fiber. A daily serving of cooked beans may lower blood cholesterol by as much as 18 percent, decreasing the risk of heart disease by more than 50 percent. In addition to high protein and fiber, the fava bean has a unique water-soluble protein that has shown a remarkable ability to scavenge free radicals, acting as an antioxidant. Try the irresistible flavors of this celebrated legume in *Foul* (Fava Bean Stew).

It's important to note that fresh fava beans can be poisonous to a very small percentage of individuals, usually those of Mediterranean descent. Favism is a rare inherited disorder of an enzyme deficiency; glucose-6-phosphate dehydrogenase (G6PD). Individuals who are G6PD-deficient can cause severe damage to red blood cells and subsequent anemia if they eat fava beans. One out of five people with this deficiency develops symptoms, such as fatigue, shortness of breath, and an irregular heartbeat, usually after eating raw or partially cooked fava beans. Several methods are used to diagnose favism, including a simple blood test.

CHICKPEAS

The nutty-flavored chickpea, also known as the garbanzo bean, has a cosmopolitan history. It's been around for thousands of years and holds a prominent place in distinguished tables from Sicily to Bombay.

Rich in protein, chickpeas are doubly useful: Immature shoots and the beans themselves are enjoyed as a vegetable. In the Middle East, chickpeas are ground with garlic and spices for a highly seasoned dip called *hummus* or formed into balls and deep-fried in tasty sandwiches called *falafel.*

When dried and ground, chickpeas can also be used as flour for sweet and savory dishes, such as *Socca,* a tender and savory crêpe from the South of France. Halva is a luscious Indian dessert pudding that can also be made with chickpea flour.

A rich source of phytosterols (the cholesterol clone), chickpeas promote heart health by decreasing the absorption of cholesterol. They're also loaded with fiber, thus increasing satiety, which may keep obesity under control by reducing overall intake.

Relish the savory flavors of this versatile legume in Falafel Sandwiches and Persian Vegetable Stew.

BLACK BEANS

The deep color of their protective black coat is a tip-off that black beans are loaded with phytochemicals. Their abundance of flavonoids has antioxidant energy to protect us against chronic diseases and the effects of aging.

If you're watching your weight, a hearty bowl of fiber-filled black bean soup is a great way to start a meal. You'll feel satisfied before you have a chance to eat a lot more. Like most legumes, black beans have protease inhibitors, compounds that are thought to suppress cancer cells and slow tumor growth.

Though generally thought of in terms of Spanish cuisine, black beans have subtle flavors that adapt easily to a variety of seasonings and cuisines. Indulge in their rich goodness with Tiny Chinese Black Bean Dumplings and Succotash Salad.

CANNELLINI BEANS

The cannellini bean is a large white bean that is sometimes referred to as the white kidney bean. Originally associated with Italian dishes, it is now used in many other cuisines. Along with other legumes, the cannellini bean contains *prebiotics,* nutrients that are used by specific strains of bacteria. When added to the diet, they promote the growth of beneficial bacteria in the intestine.

Many beans, especially white ones, contain *resistant starch,* a fermentable carbohydrate. Along with the bean's fiber contingent, resistant starch travels to the large intestine instead of being digested in the small intestine along with other carbohydrates. It then settles in the colon, where it's attacked by bacteria and fermented. This process produces a short-chain fatty acid called *butyrate,* which is thought to suppress tumor cell growth. It's been theorized that increased butyrate in the large intestine is associated with a lower incidence of colon cancer. White beans take a delicious turn in hearty and rustic *Jota* (Italian Bean and Sauerkraut Soup).

BEANS AND DIGESTION

Many of us associate beans with occasional digestive problems, especially if we don't eat them regularly. As complex carbohydrates, beans contain a variety of complex sugars, such as stachyose and raffinose, which require special enzymes to break them down. If the enzymes are absent in the digestive tract, the sugars begin to ferment, creating gas and intestinal distress.

When preparing dried beans, it is helpful to soak the beans overnight. This initiates the process of dissolving the complex sugars and thus minimizes their uncomfortable side effects. Before cooking the beans, they should be drained, rinsed, and covered with fresh water.

Supplemental enzymes that ease digestive problems are available on the market, and they can be taken just before taking your first bite of beans. Most of these enzymes cannot be added to the beans as they are cooking, because the high heat inactivates them.

PEANUTS

The peanut is a legume, not a nut. Half of the peanuts consumed in the United States are in the form of a one-hundred-year-old American recipe, peanut butter. But peanuts have been around far longer.

African families have enjoyed peanut stew for centuries, a national dish that is flavored and protein-fortified with ground peanuts. In fact, a city in the Congo, Nguba, is the origin of the peanut's nickname, *goober.* (*Nguba* is also the word for "peanut" in the Bantu language.) Peanuts have a cache of the antioxidant resveratrol, which fights heart disease by decreasing the oxidation of LDL (bad cholesterol) and preventing blood clotting. Phytosterols, especially beta-sterol, play a protective role in fighting cancer by inhibiting the growth of tumor cells. Taste a new form of peanuts in savory African Groundnut Stew.

LENTILS

A discussion of luxury foods would never include lentils; they've been considered a poor man's provision for over eight thousand years. Lentils have been revered in India and the Middle East for centuries. It's no wonder. Some of the world's greatest religions prescribe a vegetarian diet, and lentils are a great substitute for meat. They're high in protein and loaded with minerals. A ½-cup serving of cooked lentils has 20 grams of complex carbohydrates, 8 grams of dietary fiber, and a whopping 9 grams of protein. Lentils are also one of the richest natural sources of folate.

Hippocrates, the father of medicine (and an antiaging visionary), prescribed lentils to his patients with liver ailments. His foresight is legendary. Lentils contain saponins, a powerful phytochemical and antioxidant that may help to prevent cancer cells from multiplying, according to preliminary animal research. There is also evidence that lentils in the diet may contribute to improved control of blood sugar, cholesterol, and triglycerides due to their high fiber content.

Taste lentils in a new light with the bright flavors of Creamy Chickpea and Lentil Stew and Stovetop Barbecued Lentils.

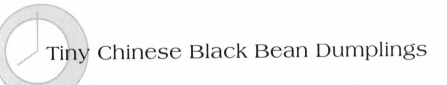

Tiny Chinese Black Bean Dumplings

Bite into these pillows of creamy black beans with a fragrant blend of Asian seasonings. They're great make-ahead hors d'oeuvres: Just pop them in a steamer for 6 minutes and they're ready to serve.

YIELD: ABOUT 30 DUMPLINGS; 6 (5-DUMPLING) SERVINGS
PREPARATION TIME: 1 HOUR

> *1 tablespoon olive oil*
> *½ cup finely chopped yellow onion*
> *2 tablespoons minced garlic*

2 tablespoons peeled, minced fresh ginger
½ cup finely shredded green cabbage
1½ cups cooked black beans or 1 (15-ounce) can, drained and rinsed
2 tablespoons low-sodium soy sauce
3 tablespoons finely chopped fresh cilantro, without stems
Salt and pepper to taste
30 round won ton wrappers (see Note, page 171)
Cornstarch for dusting

Garnish:
Cilantro sprigs

Prepare dumpling filling: Heat oil in a medium sauté pan over medium heat. Add onion and sauté until soft and transparent, about 2 minutes. Add garlic and ginger; sauté for 1 minute. Do not brown garlic.

Add cabbage and stir-fry the mixture until the cabbage is soft and wilted, about 3 minutes. Add black beans, soy sauce, and cilantro, and season with salt and pepper; cook 1 minute. Remove from heat and set aside to cool.

Place the cooled filling in the bowl of a food processor. Pulse a few times, but do not puree. You will have a chunky mixture.

Assemble dumplings: Place about 2 teaspoons of filling in the center of each won ton wrapper. Fold in half to form a half-moon, and pinch one end of the half-moon together. Using your thumb and index finger, make four or five small pleats in the front piece of dough, then pinch the other end of the dough to seal the dumpling. If necessary, brush dough with a little water to help the layers stick together.

Dust each dumpling lightly with cornstarch. Stand each dumpling so the rounded edge is upright. (The dumplings may be prepared up to this point, 8 hours in advance, and kept loosely covered and refrigerated. They may also be prepared 1 month in advance and kept tightly covered and frozen. If the dumplings are frozen, do not thaw them before cooking.)

Steam the dumplings, covered, for about 6 minutes. Garnish the dumplings with the cilantro sprigs and serve hot.

NOTE: Won ton wrappers are available in Asian markets and in the ethnic section of many supermarkets.

Black Bean Factoid: Black beans have a mildly sweet flavor and a dense texture. Black beans with rice is a staple dish in Brazil, Mexico, and the Caribbean.

Nutrient Analysis: per 5-dumpling serving

CALORIES: 195   PROTEIN: 9 grams   CARBS.: 30 grams   TOTAL FAT: 4 grams   SAT. FAT: 0 gram

POLY. FAT: 0 gram   MONO. FAT: 2 grams   CHOLES.: 4 mgs   FIBER: 4 grams   SODIUM: 432 mgs

Creamy Chickpea and Lentil Stew with Caramelized Onions

This satisfying stew is loaded with legumes, protein, and flavor. A handful of bulgur adds extra body and a lot of fiber. This recipe works well for freezing and reheating.

YIELD: 1½ QUARTS; 6 (1-CUP) SERVINGS

PREPARATION TIME: 45 MINUTES

1 medium red bell pepper
2 tablespoons olive oil
1 cup finely chopped yellow onion
1 teaspoon ground coriander
½ teaspoon ground cumin
4 cups fat-free chicken or vegetable broth
½ cup rinsed, dry yellow lentils
¼ cup coarsely ground bulgur
1½ cups cooked garbanzo beans or 1 (15-ounce) can, drained and rinsed
¼ cup chopped fresh cilantro, without stems
Salt and pepper to taste

Roast the whole red pepper under a broiler or on the stovetop, turning occasionally until the skin blisters and chars all over. Place in a bowl, cover with a lid, and let steam to loosen the skin. Carefully peel away the skin and remove the seeds. Cut pepper into medium dice and set aside.

Heat olive oil in a 3-quart saucepan over medium heat. Add onion and sauté, stirring occasionally, until light brown and caramelized, about 12 minutes. Add spices and cook until fragrant, 1 minute. Carefully add broth and bring to a boil.

Add lentils, cover, and reduce heat to low; simmer 15 minutes. Add bulgur, cover, and cook 8 minutes. Add garbanzo beans and bell pepper and simmer 2 minutes. Stir in cilantro and season with salt and pepper. Serve hot.

Lentil Factoid: One of the oldest known foods, lentils are used extensively in most parts of the world. They do not require presoaking, cook quickly, and are premier sources of protein.

Nutrient Analysis: per 1-cup serving

CALORIES: 211   PROTEIN: 13 grams   CARBS.: 27 grams   TOTAL FAT: 6 grams   SAT. FAT: 1 gram
POLY. FAT: 1 gram   MONO. FAT: 3 grams   CHOLES.: 0 mg   FIBER: 8 grams (Sol. 1 gram)
SODIUM: 117 mgs

Jota (Italian Bean and Sauerkraut Soup)

This hearty classic soup from the northern region of Italy knows many variations, though beans and sauerkraut are always included. If you have the luxury of time, the soup is best the second day, after the flavors have married. Serve with crusty bread for dipping.

YIELD: 1¾ QUARTS; 7 (1-CUP) SERVINGS
PREPARATION TIME: 30 MINUTES

2 tablespoons olive oil
1½ cups finely chopped yellow onion

4 minced garlic cloves

2 tablespoons stone-ground cornmeal

1 teaspoon yellow mustard seeds

2 cups sauerkraut, rinsed and drained

4 cups fat-free chicken or vegetable broth

1 bay leaf

1 teaspoon dried thyme

1½ cups cooked cannellini beans or 1 (15-ounce) can, drained
    and rinsed

Salt and pepper to taste

Garnish:
2 tablespoons chopped fresh Italian parsley, without stems

Heat oil in a 3-quart saucepan over medium heat. Add onions and sauté until translucent and just beginning to brown, 5 minutes. Add garlic and sauté 1 minute. Do not brown. Stir in cornmeal and mustard seeds until combined. Stir in sauerkraut and simmer 2 minutes.

Carefully add broth, bay leaf, and thyme; bring to a boil. Stir in beans and return to a boil. Reduce heat to low and simmer 5 minutes. Season with salt and pepper.

Remove bay leaf before serving. Garnish with parsley.

Cannellini Bean Factoid: This creamy white kidney bean is popular in Italian cuisine and is often pureed and flavored for creamy spreads. White beans also contain resistant starch, which may play a complementary role to soluble fiber in decreasing cholesterol, stabilizing blood sugar, and fighting cancer.

Nutrient Analysis: per 1-cup serving

CALORIES: 108   PROTEIN: 8 grams   CARBS.: 14 grams   TOTAL FAT: 2 grams   SAT. FAT: 0 gram

POLY. FAT: 0 gram   MONO. FAT: 1 gram   CHOLES.: 0 mg   FIBER: 4 grams (Sol. 2 grams)

SODIUM: 224 mgs

Persian Vegetable Stew

This flavorful stew can be varied in limitless ways. Loaded with fiber, a 1-cup serving is rich in protein, too. The recipe adapts well to experimention with different beans or greens instead of spinach.

YIELD: 1½ QUARTS; 6 (1-CUP) SERVINGS
PREPARATION TIME: 45 MINUTES

2 tablespoons olive oil
2 medium finely chopped yellow onions
3 chopped garlic cloves
1 teaspoon ground turmeric
1½ cups cooked garbanzo beans or 1 (15-ounce) can, drained
   and rinsed
1½ cups cooked cannellini beans or 1 (15-ounce) can, drained
   and rinsed
3 cups fat-free chicken or vegetable broth
8 ounces washed chopped fresh spinach leaves or 1 (8-ounce) package
   frozen chopped spinach, thawed and drained
¼ cup chopped fresh cilantro, without stems
2 tablespoons chopped fresh dill or 2 teaspoons dried
Salt and pepper to taste

Heat oil in a 3-quart saucepan over medium heat. Add onions and sauté until softened and just beginning to brown, about 5 minutes. Add garlic and cook 1 minute; do not brown garlic. Add turmeric and beans. Stir well to combine. Add broth and bring to a simmer.

Add spinach and bring to boil. Reduce heat to low and simmer about 3 minutes. Stir in fresh herbs and season with salt and pepper. Serve hot.

Bean Factoid: Canned beans are usually high in sodium. Rinsing canned beans removes as much as 40 percent of their sodium.

Nutrient Analysis: per 1-cup serving

CALORIES: 257 PROTEIN: 13 grams CARBS.: 36 grams TOTAL FAT: 7 grams SAT. FAT: 1 gram
POLY. FAT: 2 grams MONO. FAT: 4 grams CHOLES.: 0 mg FIBER: 10 grams (Sol. 2 grams)
SODIUM: 281 mgs

Succotash Salad

Succotash, a Native American word for a mixture of beans and corn, is traditionally made with lima beans. This rendition opts for black beans, though the flavor isn't compromised in this deliciously addictive salad.

YIELD: 5 CUPS; 10 (½-CUP) SERVINGS
PREPARATION TIME: 30 MINUTES

Salad:
1 tablespoon olive oil
½ cup chopped red onion
1 tablespoon minced garlic
2 cups fresh or frozen corn kernels (thawed)
1½ cups seeded, chopped tomatoes
1½ cups cooked cannellini beans or 1 (15-ounce) can, drained
   and rinsed
1½ cups cooked black beans or 1 (15-ounce) can, drained and rinsed
¼ cup chopped green onion (green and white parts)
Salt and pepper to taste

Dressing:

1 teaspoon Dijon mustard
1 teaspoon fresh lemon juice
1 minced garlic clove
1 tablespoon sorghum syrup or dark honey
¼ cup rice wine vinegar
¼ cup extra-virgin olive oil

2 tablespoons chopped fresh cilantro, without stems

Prepare salad: Heat oil in a large sauté pan over medium heat. Add onion and sauté until softened, about 3 minutes. Add garlic and sauté 1 minute. Do not brown garlic. Add corn and tomatoes; sauté for about 3 minutes. Add beans and cook 1 minute. Stir in green onion. Season with salt and pepper. Remove from heat and transfer to a large mixing bowl. Set aside.

Prepare dressing: Whisk together all the ingredients except the oil in a small nonreactive mixing bowl. Pour in olive oil in a thin stream, whisking continuously until all the oil is incorporated.

Pour dressing over salad and stir to combine. Sprinkle with cilantro.

Bean Factoid: Excellent sources of complex carbohydrates, beans contain complex sugars, too. Some of them (e.g., stachyose and raffinose) are difficult to digest and cause discomfort and gas. Add beans to your diet gradually or take a supplemental enzyme to minimize this effect.

Nutrient Analysis: per ½-cup serving

CALORIES: 162 PROTEIN: 6 grams CARBS.: 18 grams TOTAL FAT: 8 grams SAT. FAT: 1 gram
POLY. FAT: 1 gram MONO. FAT: 5 grams CHOLES.: 0 mg FIBER: 5 grams SODIUM: 25 mgs

Falafel Sandwiches

A Middle Eastern classic, *falafel* is a highly seasoned blend of chickpeas that is formed into balls or patties. Classically they are deep-fried. In this recipe they are baked for a lighter and softer falafel, but there's no compromise on the flavor. They are served in a pita bread sandwich, nestled in a bed of crispy lettuce, tomato, and cucumber. Serve them with Lemon Tahini Sauce (page 46) for an unforgettable meal.

YIELD: 10 PIECES; 5 (2-PIECE) SERVINGS
PREPARATION TIME: 30 MINUTES

Falafel:
2 teaspoons olive oil
1 cup minced onion
4 minced garlic cloves
½ teaspoon salt (optional)
1 teaspoon ground cumin
1 teaspoon ground turmeric
½ teaspoon ground coriander
1½ cups cooked garbanzo beans (chickpeas) or 1 (15-ounce) can,
*   drained and rinsed*
¼ cup chopped fresh cilantro, without stems
1 tablespoon fresh lemon juice
2 teaspoons tahini (see Note, page 46)

5 (4-inch) whole-wheat pita bread rounds or 3 (6-inch) halved rounds
Shredded lettuce, chopped cucumber, and sliced tomatoes
Lemon Tahini Sauce (page 46)

Preheat oven to 375 degrees Fahrenheit. Lightly coat a 15 x 10-inch baking sheet with olive oil cooking spray.

Heat olive oil in medium sauté pan over medium heat. Add onion and sauté until clear and translucent, about 5 minutes. Add garlic and sauté for 1 minute longer; do not brown garlic. Add cumin, turmeric, and coriander, and sauté until spices are fragrant, about 1 minute. Remove from heat.

Place chickpeas in the bowl of a food processor or a blender jar. Add onion mixture, cilantro, lemon juice, and tahini and pulse until mixture is well blended but not completely pureed. You will have about 2½ cups of chunky mixture.

Form mixture into 10 balls using a ⅛-cup scoop (2 tablespoons) per ball. Flatten each ball into a ½-inch-thick patty. Place patties on prepared baking sheet. Bake 10 minutes. Turn patties; bake another 10 minutes.

Slice each pita bread in half to form 2 pockets. Fill each half with 2 hot falafel patties, lettuce, cucumber, and tomato. Top each pocket with a dollop of sauce.

Garbanzo Bean Factoid: Also called chickpeas, garbanzos are firm, round, beige beans used extensively in Middle Eastern, Indian, and Mediterranean cuisines. One ½-cup serving has 7 grams of protein and 60 milligrams of calcium.

Nutrient Analysis: per 2 falafel patties with pita bread, lettuce, cucumber, and tomato
CALORIES: 208   PROTEIN: 9 grams   CARBS.: 34 grams   TOTAL FAT: 5 grams   SAT. FAT: 1 gram
POLY. FAT: 1 gram   MONO. FAT: 2 grams   CHOLES.: 0 mg   FIBER: 7 grams (Sol. 1 gram)
SODIUM: 176 mgs

African Groundnut Stew

In Africa, *groundnut* is the name commonly used for *peanut*. Though this popular native dish is usually prepared with chicken, soybeans are used in this version. A thick and robust stew, it's hearty enough for a main course. You can add extra broth for thinner soup. It's loaded with both protein and fiber.

YIELD: 2 QUARTS; 8 (1-CUP) SERVINGS

PREPARATION TIME: 1 HOUR

1 tablespoon extra-virgin olive oil
1 finely chopped medium red onion
1 finely chopped medium green bell pepper
½ cup chopped carrot
½ cup chopped celery
3 minced garlic cloves
2 tablespoon peeled, minced fresh ginger
1 tablespoon curry powder
2 large peeled, halved, seeded, chopped tomatoes
 (see Note, page 195) or 1 cup tomato sauce
1 bay leaf
4 cups fat-free chicken or vegetable broth
1 (12-ounce) sweet potato, peeled and cut into ½-inch dice
1½ cups cooked dried soybeans; or 1 (15-ounce) can, drained and
 rinsed; or 1½ cups cooked edamame
3 tablespoons creamy or crunchy natural peanut butter
¼ cup chopped fresh cilantro, without stems
½ pound baby spinach leaves or other fresh greens, torn into bite-size
 pieces
Salt and pepper to taste

Heat olive oil in a 4-quart saucepan or Dutch oven over medium heat. Add onion, bell pepper, carrot, and celery and sauté until soft and translucent, about 5 minutes. Add garlic, ginger, and curry powder and sauté until fragrant; do not brown garlic. Add tomatoes and bay leaf and cook, uncovered, until tomatoes are slightly reduced, about 3 minutes.

Add broth and bring mixture to a boil. Reduce heat to low. Add sweet potato and simmer for about 5 minutes. Stir in soybeans and peanut butter until combined. Cook until heated through, about 2 minutes. Stir in cilantro and spinach. Season with salt and pepper.

Peanut Factoid: Regular peanut butter contains a small amount of partially hydrogenated oil and trans fatty acids. This keeps the oil from separating out of the peanut butter, but, like harmful cholesterol, it's not something we want lingering in our bloodstreams. In natural peanut butters, which do not contain partially hydrogenated oils, the peanut oil rises to the top, but a quick stir will restore its creamy consistency.

Nutrient Analysis: per 1-cup serving

CALORIES: 185   PROTEIN: 12 grams   CARBS.: 21 grams   TOTAL FAT: 7 grams   SAT. FAT: 1 gram
POLY. FAT: 2 grams   MONO. FAT: 3 grams   CHOLES.: 0 mg   FIBER: 6 grams (Sol. 2 grams)
SODIUM: 204 mgs

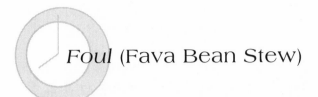

Foul (Fava Bean Stew)

F*oul* (pronounced *fūl*), a traditional morning meal in the Middle East, consists of heavily seasoned fava beans. It contains garlic, lemon juice, and olive oil; sometimes tomatoes and onions are added. This tomato-rich version is best served hot with whole-grain pita bread and slivers of green onion.

YIELD: 2 CUPS; 8 (¼-CUP) SERVINGS
PREPARATION TIME: 15 MINUTES

> 1½ cups cooked fava or broad beans or 1 (15-ounce) can),
>   drained and rinsed
> 1 tablespoon olive oil
> ½ cup chopped red onion
> 1 tablespoon minced garlic
> ½ cup chopped tomato
> 1 teaspoon ground cumin
> ½ cup tomato sauce
> 1 tablespoon fresh lime (or lemon) juice
> 1 tablespoon chopped fresh Italian parsley, without stems
> 1 tablespoon chopped fresh cilantro, without stems
> Salt and pepper to taste

Garnish:
1 finely chopped green onion (green and white parts)

Place half of the beans in a small mixing bowl and mash with a fork until chunky but not smooth. Set aside.

Heat oil in a large sauté pan over medium-high heat. Add onion and sauté until soft and translucent, about 3 minutes. Add garlic and sauté 1 minute; do not brown garlic. Add tomato and cumin and simmer 2 minutes. Add tomato sauce, mashed beans, and remaining beans, and cook 1 minute.

Stir in lime juice, parsley, and cilantro until combined. Remove from heat and season with salt and pepper. Transfer to a serving bowl and garnish with green onion.

> NOTE: Canned and dried fava beans can be found in Middle Eastern markets or in the ethnic section of many supermarkets. Fresh fava beans are seasonal; if unavailable, black beans can be used.
>
> *Fava Bean Factoid:* Fava or broad beans contain a compound called *L-dopa*. People with Parkinson's disease may have symptoms aggravated by fava bean consumption, and people taking medications containing L-dopa should be aware that broad bean consumption might increase L-dopa levels excessively. Therefore, Parkinson's disease patients should speak with a doctor before adding fava beans to their diet.

Nutrient Analysis: per ¼-cup serving

CALORIES: 87 PROTEIN: 4 grams CARBS.: 14 grams TOTAL FAT: 2 grams SAT. FAT: 0 gram
POLY. FAT: 0 gram MONO. FAT: 1 gram CHOLES.: 0 mg FIBER: 3 grams SODIUM: 122 mgs

Socca (Chickpea Crêpes)

These delicate nutty crêpes are a specialty in the South of France. They're delicious topped with Creamy Hummus (page 110) or *Baba Ghanouj* (Roasted Eggplant Purée) (page 73) or served with a steamy bowl of soup or stew.

YIELD: 20 (6-INCH) CRÊPES; 10 (2-CRÊPE) SERVINGS
PREPARATION TIME: 40 MINUTES

1½ cups chickpea flour (see Note, page 183)
½ cup sorghum flour

½ teaspoon salt
½ teaspoon mustard powder
¼ teaspoon ground ginger
1¾ cups unflavored soymilk
1 tablespoon olive oil

Mix flours, salt, and spices in a medium mixing bowl. Add soymilk and beat with a whisk until smooth. Beat in olive oil. Allow batter to sit for 20 minutes. (There will be about 2½ cups of batter.)

Heat a small nonstick skillet or nonstick crêpe pan over medium heat. Coat lightly with olive oil spray. Add about ⅛ cup (2 tablespoons) batter to the pan, tilting it so the batter thins out to a 6-inch circle. Cook about 30 seconds, until the crêpe is golden brown on the bottom. Using a spatula, flip crêpe over, and cook 10 to 15 seconds. Transfer crêpe to a plate and keep covered. Repeat with remaining batter, placing a sheet of waxed paper or parchment between crêpes to prevent sticking, to make about 20 crêpes. Serve hot.

NOTE: Chickpea flour is available in the ethnic section of some supermarkets and also in East Indian markets. See Shopping Sources (pages 231–32).

Chickpea Factoid: One-half cup chickpea flour contains 10 grams of protein and no gluten. In Indian markets, chickpea flour is called *besan*.

Nutrient Analysis: per 2-crêpe serving
CALORIES: 95 PROTEIN: 4 grams CARBS.: 13 grams TOTAL FAT: 3 grams SAT. FAT: 0 gram
POLY. FAT: 0.5 gram MONO. FAT: 1 gram CHOLES.: 0 mg FIBER: 1 gram SODIUM: 122 mgs

Stovetop Barbecued Lentils

Quick and easy, this barbecue favorite is absolutely addictive. A great make-ahead dish for a potluck or a picnic, it's loaded with fiber.

YIELD: 2 QUARTS; 8 (½-CUP) SERVINGS
PREPARATION TIME: 40 MINUTES

1 tablespoon olive oil
1 cup chopped red onion
1 tablespoon minced garlic
2 teaspoons chili powder
1 teaspoon mustard powder
2 cups fat-free chicken or vegetable broth
¾ cup tomato sauce
3 tablespoons balsamic vinegar
1 tablespoon Dijon mustard
2 tablespoons sorghum syrup or dark honey
1½ cups rinsed yellow lentils
Salt and pepper to taste

Heat olive oil in a 2-quart saucepan over medium heat. Add onion and sauté until softened and translucent, about 3 minutes. Add garlic and spices and sauté until fragrant, about 1 minute; do not brown garlic.

Add broth, tomato sauce, vinegar, mustard, sorghum syrup, and lentils. Stir well and bring to a boil. Reduce heat to low, cover, and simmer until lentils are tender but intact, about 30 minutes. Lentil cooking times vary. If necessary, add an additional ¼ cup water and simmer 5 minutes longer if lentils are not tender. Season with salt and pepper.

Lentil Factoid: Lentils are very high in folic acid. One cup of cooked lentils provides 90 percent of the daily recommended intake for adults.

Nutrient Analysis: per ½-cup serving

CALORIES: 159   PROTEIN: 11 grams   CARBS.: 28 grams   TOTAL FAT: 1 gram   SAT. FAT: 0 gram

POLY. FAT: 0 gram   MONO. FAT: 0 gram   CHOLES.: 0 mg   FIBER: 8 grams (Sol. 1 gram)

SODIUM: 54 mgs

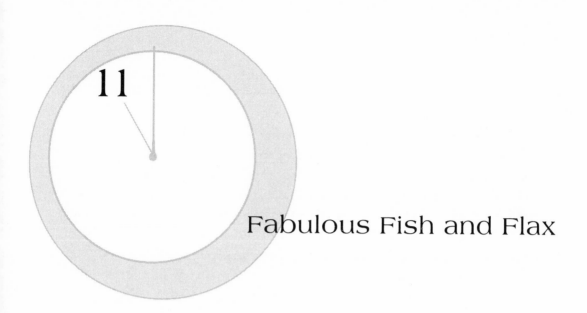

11

Fabulous Fish and Flax

There are fats with antiaging properties that benefit the entire human body—the omega-3 fatty acids. Along with the omega-6 fatty acids, they are also vital to human life, and, for that reason, they're both called *essential fatty acids* (EFAs). A balanced intake of these EFAs offers optimal health benefits. But most of us eat too many omega-6s, which can have pro-aging effects ranging from inflammatory disorders to an increased risk for heart attack, stroke, and cancer. A diet rich in omega-3 foods can restore the balance and may even reverse disease processes.

FISH

The greatest treasures of the sea are not buried. Some of Mother Nature's unrivaled riches, including plump and glistening salmon, mackerel, and herring, are cloistered in frosty ocean waters. What distinguishes these piscine creatures from other fish has everything to do with their polar habitat. The thick layer of fatty insulation they wear harbors potent, antiaging essential fats, called *omega-3 fatty acids,* which are not produced in the body but are obtained only through diet.

Does this mean eating *more* of this fat has remarkable antiaging benefits? Absolutely. Certain fats alter the production of chemical messengers called *hormones.* Programmed to travel to specific parts of the body, a hormone's job is to elicit a particular response. Omega-3s control the production of several beneficial hormones that promote a diverse range of anti-aging functions that affect heart health, brain function, cancer risk, and more. Here's how. The brain requires a high concentration of omega-3s for normal function. When levels are lower than optimal, it is believed that the function of some brain cells is compromised. This can lead to losses of vision, concentration, attention, or memory—many of the problems associated with aging.

Caribbean Salmon Croquettes or a steaming bowl of Spicy Fish Stew loaded with omega-3s might help you beat the blues or jog your memory. But that's not all. Omega-3 fatty acids promote heart health. Some of their benevolence includes:

- decreasing levels of harmful cholesterol and triglycerides,
- decreasing blood-clotting factors,
- increasing beneficial relaxation in arteries and blood vessels, which facilitates the flow of oxygen, and
- promoting blood pressure control.

With heart disease weighing in as the number-one killer in the United States, these benefits are not to be ignored. Whereas *restriction* is the key to optimal heart health with saturated fats, the omega-3 fats are *required.*

Centuries ago, our ancestors' diet consisted of game and fish that fed on wild green forage and algae whose chlorophyll-containing cells are premier sources of omega-3s. As civilization has evolved, our diet has relied less and less upon these sources, resulting in a general deficit of omega-3s in our diet and in our bodies. It's time to add them back. Regular consumption of wild cold-water fish, such as salmon, mackerel, and herring, can bolster your reserves. Three-Fish Etouffée with Baby Artichokes and Spicy Tomato Basil or Pan-Roasted Salmon with Wilted Chard and Tomato-Mint Raita are delicious ways to boost your omega-3s and turn back the clock.

We're each given a genetic map that determines the amount of omega-3s found in the nervous system, the brain, the eyes, the adrenal glands, and the sex glands, but high levels of stress, alcohol, nicotine, and caffeine and the aging process itself work against our bodies' reserves. Our diet holds the answer.

Omega-3s have anti-inflammatory properties, too. Eating more fish can minimize the pain and discomfort associated with arthritis, rheumatism, and lupus. Omega-3s inhibit many factors that contribute to the discomfort associated with inflammatory diseases. Regular intake of fish is also associated with higher levels of pulmonary function. In addition, some studies have linked fish oil to the prevention of certain kidney disorders. The list goes on. Omega-3s can also counteract the sometimes harmful effects of certain hormones, such as those that contribute to tumor growth in a variety of cancers. Emerging research indicates that omega-3s can reduce the risk of developing cancers of the breast and prostate by inhibiting the synthesis of harmful hormones that may promote tumor growth. Though there are more human studies to be done, we do know that the amount and type of dietary fatty acids can profoundly affect life span in lab animals.

According to her research on increased omega-3 consumption, Alexandra Richardson, senior neuroscience research fellow at Britain's University of Oxford, comments that "there are hardly any negative side-effects, only nice cosmetic ones such as shiny hair, strong nails, and healthy-looking skin." Chicken and eggs are also potential sources of omega-3 fats, since some chickens eat plants containing these fatty acids. Free-range chickens are the most reliable sources. Omega-3–enriched eggs are another option. Supplementing the diet of egg-laying hens with ground flaxseed yields eggs with higher concentrations of omega-3s. The cholesterol and total fat levels of these eggs are similar to those of nonenriched eggs.

FLAX

Flax is stellar plant source of omega-3 fatty acids. The flax plant is the king of utility: Its fibers are woven for linen cloth, and some of its oils, such as linseed, have industrial forms. Flaxseed oil and ground flaxseeds provide an edible form of omega-3 fatty acids called *alpha-linolenic acid* (ALA). In the body, ALA converts to the form of omega-3s found in fish oil, though the process is much slower. Still, ALA has similar antiaging benefits related to heart health and cancer, and it promotes laxation. ALA is also found in canola oil, soybean oil, and walnuts, but flax yields the highest concentration of ALA.

In addition to omega-3s, flaxseed contains phytochemical lignans. During digestion, flax lignans are converted to a weak form of estrogen thought to bind to estrogen receptors and inhibit the growth of estrogen-stimulated breast cancer. This action reduces the growth rate of cancer cells, including those in estrogen-sensitive tumors, especially of the breast and uterus. This plant estrogen activity also appears to simulate some of estrogen's benefits, such as promoting bone density and fighting osteoporosis. It also supports heart health by helping to lower cholesterol. Lignans are removed from flaxseed during refining. This means that flaxseed oil contains no lignans, although some manufacturers add them back to the refined oil.

Because they can be found in fish, chicken, nuts, and seeds, omega-3 fatty acids can easily be added to your diet. Get a jump-start on your day with Whole-Grain Flaxjacks or Lemony French Toast.

Three-Fish Étouffée with Baby Artichokes and Spicy Tomato Broth

Etouffée is a spicy Cajun stew traditionally made with crawfish, vegetables, and a dark roux. A classic etouffée is served over rice; try it over nutty whole grains for a satisfying meal with staying power.

YIELD: 2¾ QUARTS; 8 (1⅓-CUP) SERVINGS
PREPARATION TIME: 1 HOUR

¼ cup olive oil
¼ cup unbleached all-purpose flour
1 cup chopped yellow onion
⅓ cup chopped red bell pepper
¼ cup celery, cut into ½-inch dice
½ cup peeled carrot, cut into ½-inch dice
2 tablespoons minced garlic
1 cup peeled, halved, seeded, chopped tomatoes (see Note, page 195)
    or 1 cup tomato sauce
2 teaspoons finely chopped fresh oregano or ½ teaspoon dried
1 teaspoon red pepper flakes (optional)

1 cup red wine or water

4 cups fat-free fish, chicken, or vegetable broth

9 ounces fresh artichoke hearts, quartered, or 1 (9-ounce) package
*   frozen artichoke hearts, thawed and quartered lengthwise*

1 small bay leaf

2 ounces fresh shiitake mushrooms, stemmed and caps sliced (about
*   1 cup)*

1½ pounds assorted boneless fish fillets (such as salmon, mackerel,
*   tuna), cut into 1-inch cubes*

¼ cup chopped fresh parsley, without stems

1½ tablespoons finely grated lemon peel

Salt and pepper to taste

Heat oil in a 4-quart pot or large Dutch oven over medium heat. Stir in flour and cook, stirring constantly, until flour is lightly browned.

Add onion, bell pepper, celery, and carrot and cook until tender. Add garlic, tomato, oregano, and red pepper flakes (if using); simmer 1 minute longer. Add wine and bring to a boil. Reduce heat and simmer until the wine has reduced by half, about 5 minutes. The mixture will be slightly thickened.

Stir in broth and bring to a boil. Reduce heat. Add artichoke hearts, bay leaf, and mushrooms and simmer 2 minutes. Add fish; cook, stirring gently, until just opaque, about 4 minutes. Stir in parsley and lemon peel. Season with salt and pepper. Serve hot.

Omega-3 Factoid: The brilliant orange, red, and pink colors of salmon come from a substance called *astaxanthin,* a pigment from the carotenoid family that possesses strong antioxidant activity.

Nutrient Analysis: per 1⅓-cup serving

CALORIES: 346 PROTEIN: 26 grams CARBS.: 28 grams TOTAL FAT: 12 grams SAT. FAT: 2 grams
POLY. FAT: 2 grams MONO. FAT: 7 grams CHOLES.: 38 mgs FIBER: 7 grams (Sol. 2 grams)
SODIUM: 159 mgs

Caribbean Salmon Croquettes

Croquettes are the perfect answer for that salmon left over from last night's barbecue. These delicious morsels can be served as hors d'oeuvres, with a salad course, or as an entrée. They lend themselves to being made ahead, too.

YIELD: 16 CROQUETTES; 4 (4-CROQUETTE) SERVINGS
PREPARATION TIME: ABOUT 1 HOUR

2 tablespoons olive oil
1 tablespoon unbleached all-purpose flour
½ cup unflavored soymilk
¾ cup finely chopped red onion
2 tablespoons peeled, minced fresh ginger
1½ teaspoons minced garlic
1 teaspoon ground coriander
¾ teaspoon ground cumin
½ cup peeled, halved, seeded, chopped tomatoes (see Note, page 195)
12 ounces boneless, skinless cooked salmon (16 ounces as purchased
    raw, boneless, skinless)
¼ cup chopped fresh cilantro, without stems
1 tablespoon fresh lime juice
1 tablespoon grated lime peel
Salt and pepper to taste
¾ cup unseasoned panko bread crumbs (see Note, page 102) or plain
    dry bread crumbs
Olive oil cooking spray

Garnish:
1 lime, cut into 8 wedges

Lightly coat a 15 x 10-inch baking sheet with olive oil cooking spray. Position a rack in bottom third of oven.

Heat 1 tablespoon of the olive oil in a 1-quart saucepan over medium heat. Whisk in flour and cook 1 minute. Stir in soymilk and cook, whisking constantly, to make a thick cream sauce. Remove from heat and set aside to cool.

Heat remaining 1 tablespoon oil in a small sauté pan over medium heat. Add onion and sauté until softened but not browned. Add ginger and garlic. Sauté 1 minute; do not brown garlic. Add coriander and cumin, then tomatoes; sauté 1 minute. Transfer to a medium bowl to cool.

Add salmon, cilantro, lime juice, lime peel, and cream sauce to the onion mixture. Season with salt and pepper. Mixture should stick together but be dry enough to form croquettes. (If mixture is too wet, add 1 or 2 tablespoons of additional bread crumbs to absorb excess liquid.)

Place bread crumbs on a large plate. Using a ⅛-cup scoop or 2-tablespoon measure for uniformity, form mixture into about 16 round croquettes. Place croquettes on a plate. Carefully roll each of the croquettes in crumbs, pressing to adhere. Transfer to another plate. (Can be prepared up to 4 hours ahead. Cover and chill.)

Preheat oven to 425 degrees Fahrenheit. Transfer croquettes to the prepared baking sheet. Coat croquettes lightly with olive oil spray.

Place the baking sheet on the bottom shelf of the oven and bake about 6 minutes. Turn croquettes with a spatula to brown the opposite side. Bake about 5 minutes, or until croquettes are lightly golden. Serve with lime wedges.

Omega-3 Factoid: The amount and composition of fat in fish vary not only between but also within species and is dependent on season, feeding grounds, and water temperature among other factors.

Nutrient Analysis: per 4-croquette serving

CALORIES: 350 PROTEIN: 27 grams CARBS.: 25 grams TOTAL FAT: 14 grams SAT. FAT: 2 grams

POLY. FAT: 4 grams MONO. FAT: 8 grams CHOLES.: 62 mgs FIBER: 2 grams SODIUM: 241 mgs

Pan-Roasted Salmon with
Wilted Chard and Tomato-Mint Raita

Raita is a classic yogurt-based condiment typically served with East Indian food. The cool tang of the yogurt and the fresh crunch of minced vegetables are intended to balance the spiciness of curry, as in this easy yet elegant salmon dish. Serve with Caribbean Sweet Potatoes (page 182) for an extraordinary feast.

YIELD: 4 SERVINGS

PREPARATION TIME: 50 MINUTES

Tomato-Mint Raita:

2 peeled, seeded, diced plum tomatoes (see Note, page 195)

1 cup seeded, diced cucumber

1 cup plain fat-free yogurt or soy yogurt (which will result in a slightly sweeter taste)

2 tablespoons minced fresh mint leaves, without stems

½ teaspoon ground mustard

½ teaspoon red pepper flakes (optional)

Pinch ground cumin

Salt and pepper to taste

Pan-Roasted Salmon:

2 tablespoons peeled, minced fresh ginger

1 tablespoon curry powder

Salt and pepper to taste

4 (3-ounce) pieces boneless, skinless salmon fillet

2 teaspoons olive oil

2 tablespoons chopped shallot

½ cup fat-free chicken or vegetable broth

Wilted Chard:
1 teaspoon olive oil
1 large bunch torn Swiss chard leaves, without stems
2 tablespoons fat-free chicken or vegetable broth
Salt and pepper to taste

Prepare raita: Combine tomatoes, cucumber, yogurt, mint, mustard, red pepper flakes (if using), and cumin in a small bowl. Season with salt and pepper. Set aside to allow flavors to blend.

Prepare salmon: Stir together ginger and curry powder and season with salt and pepper. Pat spice mixture onto top side of each salmon piece. (Salmon can be prepared up to 12 hours ahead and allowed to marinate before cooking.)

Heat oil in a nonstick skillet over medium heat until hot but not smoking. Add salmon, spice side down, and cook, covered, about 5 minutes. Turn salmon over and cook, covered, until just cooked through, about 2 minutes. Transfer salmon to a dinner plate.

Pour off any excess oil from pan. Add shallot to skillet and sauté 30 seconds. Stir in chicken broth and boil until reduced by half. Pour pan sauce over salmon. Keep warm.

Prepare chard: While salmon is cooking, heat oil in a large sauté pan over medium-high heat. Add chard and broth. Cover and cook until greens wilt, stirring occasionally, about 3 minutes. Uncover and cook until juices thicken slightly, about 2 minutes. Season with salt and pepper.

Place wilted greens on plate with salmon. Serve ½ cup raita with each portion.

NOTE: Remove stem and core from each tomato with a small knife. Make an x-shape cut on the bottom of each tomato. Submerge tomatoes in boiling water for 30 seconds. Remove immediately and transfer to ice water. Remove from ice water and slip off loosened skins. Cut each tomato in half and remove seeds with a spoon.

Salmon Factoid: Fish such as salmon, tuna, and mackerel are high in omega-3s because they feed on plankton, an organism that provides the fish and, ultimately, humans with the fatty acids they need.

Nutrient Analysis: per serving

CALORIES: 213   PROTEIN: 24 grams   CARBS.: 11 grams   TOTAL FAT: 9 grams   SAT. FAT: 2 grams

POLY. FAT: 2 grams   MONO. FAT: 4 grams   CHOLES.: 40 mgs   FIBER: 2 grams   SODIUM: 226 mgs

Salmon Charmoula

Charmoula is a fragrant and spicy sauce commonly found in Moroccan food stalls and served with fried fish. It's delicious with poached salmon, too. Serve with Casbah Bulgur (page 150).

YIELD: 4 SERVINGS

PREPARATION TIME: 30 MINUTES

½ teaspoon ground coriander

¼ teaspoon ground pepper

¼ teaspoon ground cumin

¼ teaspoon crumbled saffron threads (optional)

3 teaspoons olive oil

1 cup finely chopped red onion

2 tablespoons minced Preserved Lemon peel (page 48) or

2 tablespoons grated lemon peel

4 (3-ounce) pieces boneless, skinless salmon fillet

¼ cup white wine

2 tablespoons chopped fresh cilantro, without stems

Salt and pepper to taste

Prepare Charmoula: Place spices in a small mixing bowl. Set aside. Heat 2 teaspoons of the olive oil in a medium sauté pan over medium-high heat. Add onion and sauté until soft and translucent, about 4 minutes. Add spice mixture and sauté until richly fragrant, about 1 minute. Remove from heat and stir in lemon peel. Transfer to a small mixing bowl and set aside.

Return same pan to medium-high heat. Add remaining 1 teaspoon olive oil and heat until hot but not smoking. Add salmon and cook about 4 minutes. Turn salmon over and cook until just opaque, about 2 minutes. Transfer salmon to a dinner plate.

Pour off any excess oil from pan. Stir in white wine and boil until reduced by half. Stir in onion mixture and simmer until heated through. Stir in chopped cilantro and season with salt and pepper.

Top each salmon fillet with charmoula sauce and serve.

Omega-3 Factoid: There are several different species of salmon, all of which vary in fat content. Chinook has the highest fat content, and pink has the lowest.

Nutrient Analysis: per serving

CALORIES: 172   PROTEIN: 21 grams   CARBS.: 5 grams   TOTAL FAT: 7 grams   SAT. FAT: 1 gram
POLY. FAT: 1 gram   MONO. FAT: 4 grams   CHOLES.: 47 mgs   FIBER: 1 gram   SODIUM: 52 mgs

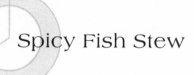

Spicy Fish Stew

The character of this savory stew depends on the fish you select. Whichever you choose, the intriguing blend of flavors results in a dish that is elegant in its simplicity.

YIELD: 1½ QUARTS; 6 (1-CUP) SERVINGS
PREPARATION TIME: 40 MINUTES

1 tablespoon olive oil
1 cup finely chopped yellow onion
1 cup finely chopped green bell pepper
1 cup peeled, halved, seeded, chopped tomatoes (see Note, page 195)
1½ teaspoons ground coriander
½ teaspoon ground cumin

4 cups fat-free chicken, fish, or vegetable broth

*1 pound boneless, skinless fish fillets (salmon, tuna, or mackerel), cut
   into ¾-inch pieces*

2 tablespoons tahini (see Note, page 46)

*1 tablespoon finely chopped Preserved Lemon peel (page 48) or grated
   lemon peel*

¼ cup finely chopped fresh cilantro, without stems

Heat olive oil in a 3-quart saucepan over medium heat. Add onion and bell pepper and sauté until soft but not browned, about 5 minutes. Add tomatoes and sauté 3 minutes. Stir in spices and simmer 1 minute.

Carefully pour in broth and bring mixture to a boil. Add fish. When mixture returns to a boil, reduce heat to low and simmer until fish is cooked through, 3 minutes.

Stir in tahini, lemon peel, and cilantro. Serve hot.

Fish Factoid: Few foods naturally contain vitamin D; tuna, salmon, and mackerel are key exceptions. A 3- to 4-ounce portion of any one of these fish can meet or even exceed the recommended daily intake for adults.

Nutrient Analysis: per 1-cup serving

CALORIES: 264   PROTEIN: 35 grams   CARBS.: 10 grams   TOTAL FAT: 9 grams   SAT. FAT: 1 gram
POLY. FAT: 2 grams   MONO. FAT: 4 grams   CHOLES.: 51 mgs   FIBER: 3 grams   SODIUM: 220 mgs

Whole-Grain Flaxjacks

In addition to their antiaging attributes, whole grains add texture and flavor to any recipe. Flaxseed contains powerful omega-3s. Cook your flaxjacks over moderate heat so they don't burn; the natural flaxseed oils make them brown more quickly. Serve hot with Warm Blueberry Compote (page 37) or Cranberry Spice Jam (page 33).

YIELD: 16 (4-INCH) PANCAKES; 8 (2-PANCAKE) SERVINGS
PREPARATION TIME: 30 MINUTES

½ cup stone-ground cornmeal
½ cup whole-wheat flour
½ cup unbleached all-purpose flour
2 tablespoons flaxseed meal (see Note, page 200)
1½ teaspoons baking powder
½ teaspoon salt
1¾ cups unflavored soymilk
1 large egg
1 large egg white
2 tablespoons olive oil
2 tablespoons sorghum syrup or dark honey

Combine dry ingredients in a large mixing bowl. Set aside. Combine remaining ingredients in a blender or whisk together in a small mixing bowl until smooth.

Make a well in center of dry ingredients. Pour liquid mixture into well; stir just until combined. Allow batter to rest 30 minutes or overnight in the refrigerator. Add additional soymilk, if needed, to obtain a batter with the consistency of thick cream.

Heat a nonstick griddle or skillet over medium heat. Lightly coat griddle with olive oil spray, if necessary.

For each pancake, pour scant ¼ cup batter onto hot griddle. Cook pancakes until puffed and dry around edges. Turn and cook the other side until golden brown.

NOTE: In a clean spice grinder, grind whole flaxseeds to the consistency of cornmeal. If not ground, or chewed well, the whole seed passes through the body intact, and you miss out on all of its benefits. When ground, flaxseeds are light reddish-brown flakes, similar to wheat bran. One-third cup of flaxseed yields about ½ cup of flaxseed meal.

Flaxseed Factoid: Make flaxseed part of your diet, because the seeds contain omega-3 fatty acids, fiber, and lignans.

Nutrient Analysis: per 2-pancake serving

CALORIES: 172 PROTEIN: 6 grams CARBS.: 23 grams TOTAL FAT: 7 grams SAT. FAT: 1 gram
POLY. FAT: 2 grams MONO. FAT: 3 grams CHOLES.: 27 mgs FIBER: 4 grams SODIUM: 217 mgs

Lemony French Toast

This recipe was inspired by Frank Canez, executive chef of Canyon Ranch at the Venetian in Las Vegas. Serve with Warm Blueberry Compote (page 37), Cranberry Spice Jam (page 33), or fresh fruit.

YIELD: 4 SERVINGS
PREPARATION TIME: 30 MINUTES

4 (1-inch-thick) slices whole-grain bread
4 tablespoons sugar-free jam or fruit spread
1 cup unflavored soymilk
2 tablespoons ground flaxseed (see Note below)
1 tablespoon sorghum syrup or dark honey
1 teaspoon pure vanilla extract
1 teaspoon grated lemon peel
Pinch salt

Place bread slices on a level work surface and make a horizontal lengthwise pocket in each by cutting to within ¼ inch of opposite side. Spoon 1 tablespoon jam into each opening and gently press closed.

Combine soymilk, flaxseed, sorghum syrup, vanilla, lemon peel, and salt in a blender jar. Puree until smooth. Pour mixture into a small shallow pan. Arrange bread slices in the milk mixture in a single layer, turning once.

Lightly coat a large nonstick skillet with olive oil cooking spray and heat skillet over medium heat. Transfer bread slices to skillet and cook until golden and crisp, about 4 minutes on each side. Transfer French toast to 4 serving plates. Serve hot.

Flax Factoid: Flaxseed is the richest dietary source of lignans, plant estrogens that have shown promise as a cancer preventive. The concentration of this beneficial substance is approximately 800 times higher in flaxseed than in other grains, nuts, and seeds.

Nutrient Analysis: per 1-slice serving

CALORIES: 139   PROTEIN: 5 grams   CARBS.: 32 grams   TOTAL FAT: 4 grams   SAT. FAT: 0 gram

POLY. FAT: 2 grams   MONO. FAT: 1 gram   CHOLES.: 0 mg   FIBER: 8 grams   SODIUM: 93 mgs

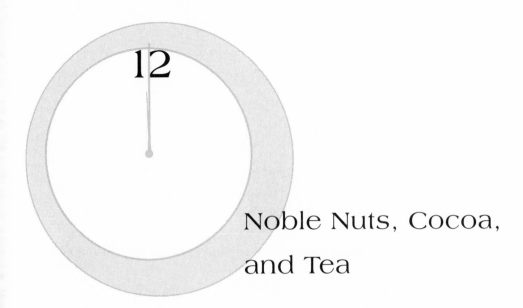

12

Noble Nuts, Cocoa, and Tea

Since the Middle Ages, nuts, cocoa, and tea have changed world patterns of trade, travel, and eating. Together, they can compose the finale to a great meal. Apart, their distinctive aromas, flavors, and textures offer myriad culinary possibilities. They've withstood the test of time; and the latest news heralds a world of healthy new reasons why they won't be going away any time soon.

NUTS

Walnuts, almonds, pine nuts, pecans, Brazil nuts—just a smattering of these crunchy nuggets can make or break a recipe. There's no easier way to revive a blasé dish than to sprinkle it with crispy toasted nuts. Toss them on cereal, salad, or dessert. Adding nuts gives a dish sensory appeal by enhancing both texture and flavor.

Nuts are a welcome antiaging bonus, too. In conjunction with a diet of fresh fruits and vegetables, lean protein, and whole grains, they provide protection from heart disease and potential reduction in blood pressure. For years, we've considered them forbidden fruit, knowing they're high in fat. However, they're also rich in protein, and the fats we thought were taboo are actually quite good, because many nuts contain essential fats such as omega-3s. And essential fats are just that—essential.

The colossal Brazil nut makes a long journey to our pantries. This is one cash crop that we haven't been able to cultivate outside of its native Amazon home. This means that a demand for Brazil nuts encourages preservation of their rain-forest habitats, but that's not the only reason to enjoy them. Brazil nuts are a powerhouse of selenium, a mighty antioxidant. One solitary Brazil nut exceeds the daily requirement for this benevolent antioxidant micronutrient.

The fats that nuts contain have cholesterol-lowering effects. Alpha-linolenic acid (ALA), particularly in walnuts, converts to omega-3s, which promote decreased levels of harmful cholesterol. Another problem leading to heart disease is artery-clogging plaque, which may result from increased stickiness of the body's clotting cells. Called *platelets,* these cells meander throughout the bloodstream. Their function is to form a clot, should bleeding occur. But too much stickiness is dangerous; it can damage the walls of blood vessels, and random clots can initiate a stroke or heart attack. Omega-3s keep *platelet aggregation,* or stickiness, in check. They also are thought to increase beneficial relaxation in arteries and blood vessels, which facilitates greater oxygen transport. Stop your clock and indulge in nutty benevolence with Banana-Caramel "Ice Cream" with Toasted Walnuts, Nutty Tomato Pesto, or Grilled Chicken with Walnut and Pomegranate Sauce.

COCOA

The sight or scent of this velvety rich concoction can actually trigger a mouth-watering response. And chocolate craving can be ferocious. Addicts have been known to tear through their pantries in search of a bar, morsel, or chip. Though it may *seem* psychological, cravings are real and are physical; we to need pay attention to how they affect our bodies.

Our nerve cells speak to us by releasing chemicals called *neurotransmitters.* We are probably most familiar with the "feel good" messenger, *serotonin.* Neurotransmitters send messages from one nerve cell to another, determining what we think, feel, do, and eat. If serotonin is low, we crave sweets. And carbohydrate foods, pasta, bread, desserts raise our serotonin levels, making us feel better and reducing our cravings.

If we took a poll on highly craved "favorites," chocolate would be *número uno.* One creamy bite not only fulfills a longing for its rich flavor but also satisfies a desire for "feel good" chemicals such as dopamine and serotonin. Chocolate's caffeine delivers an energy burst, and its fat promotes satiety. Its taste is heavenly and hinged on pleasant memories for most of us. But how does a confection like chocolate fit the antiaging picture? It's in the beans. The cocoa bean is a legume, and, prior to processing, it is remarkably rich in flavonoids. But, like fruits, vegetables, and whole grains, chocolate is refined via a process that affects its nutrient profile. And though type of bean, growing region, and farming techniques also affect the cocoa bean's nutrient content, the way it is processed has the most profound impact.

Before roasting, cocoa beans are fermented and their flavors allowed to develop. Though actual processing methods vary and are usually proprietary secrets, many manufacturers add alkali to the cocoa beans. This process is also known as *dutching,* named after after the Dutch chocolatier Conrad J. van Houten, who is credited with inventing the process. The addition of alkali results in several changes, among them a consistent end product in terms of flavor, color, and texture. It also results in a powder that dissolves more readily than nonalkalized or natural cocoa, but the alkalization step changes the flavor and reduces the residual chocolate's antioxidant flavonoid content.

Research in this area is ongoing. It is safe to say that natural cocoa powders have higher antioxidant levels, but multiple processing factors such as roasting temperature and the blend of beans create a complicated equation. The best cocoa powder for health benefits remains to be seen. So what are the antiaging attributes of our favorite flavor? Two of cocoa's flavonoids are epicatechin and procyanidin, phytochemicals that suppress multiple activities that lead to cardiovascular disease by inhibiting the development of blood platelets or clotting factors and thus helping reduce heart disease. They are also responsible for blood vessel dilation, thus promoting blood flow and reducing the risk of heart disease.

Procyanidin also bolsters immune function. This is accomplished by altering hormone or eicosanoid production to favor decreased platelet activation. Additionally, cocoa contains catechins (usually associated with green tea) that achieve a similar response. Indulge your cravings, increase your oxidative balance, and lower your risk of heart disease with Mexican Hot Chocolate or *Caponata.*

TEA

They're not exactly leafy greens, but tea leaves are stepping out of the cup and into sauce-pans in savvy kitchens. Savored for centuries, tea is known as a restorative drink with a bevy of flavors, but we rarely consider it when we think of recipes, a situation that's about to change. For centuries, tea leaves have been plucked from plants and steeped in fresh boiling water to render a soothing and familiar drink. Whether we're seeking a simple warmer-upper, a caffeine pick-me-up, or a ceremonial sip, tea is universally perceived as a beverage. It's time to step outside the box and explore its culinary prospects. But first, let's look at its antiaging phenomenon.

Green or black, tea is grown from the same basic plant. Like cocoa, tea contains a re-markable reserve of antioxidants, the concentration of which is dependent on a variety of factors, most notably its processing. The distinction between green and black tea is fer-mentation. Fermented tea leaves are black, a result of oxidized enzymes in the leaf. Green tea, on the other hand, is exposed to high temperatures immediately after harvesting, which stops fermentation in its tracks and preserves the green pigment.

Though it was originally thought that fermentation resulted in lower antioxidant activity in black tea than in green, the difference is now thought to be qualitative rather than quantitative. The flavonoids are *different.* Predominant flavonoids in green tea are epigallocatechin and epicatechin gallate, which have an abundance of antiaging power. In addition to a powerful antioxidant capacity, they boast cardioprotective benefits, including decreased cholesterol absorption, decreased platelet activity, and reduced oxidation of LDL cholesterol.

Green tea's flavonoids also appear to have an antagonistic action toward cancer cells, suppressing their activities in all stages of development, including carcinogen activation. They have been shown to be most protective against stomach and colon cancers. Black tea contains theaflavins and thearubigens, which are other forms of catechins. In addition to their antioxidant bang, they provide rich flavor and color to black tea. A growing body of evidence indicates that black tea may provide protection against the type of skin cancers caused by ultraviolet radiation. Green tea provides some of the same benefits, although they are not as pronounced. Many of the antioxidants of the tea plant are thought to have both antibacterial and antiviral properties. It is believed that they suppress the formation of cavity-causing plaque by killing the bacteria themselves. Green tea also contains natural fluorine, which further helps to prevent cavities.

Because green and black tea leaves originate from the same plant, their caffeine levels are about the same. Any difference in caffeine is a result of the brewing process. Tea bags contain broken tea leaves of smaller size and greater surface area, so they produce an infusion with more caffeine than loose tea. Black tea is usually brewed for a longer period than green tea, resulting in stronger flavor development and higher caffeine content.

Asians have cooked with tea for centuries, smoking crispy duck over fragrant tea leaves and infusing its unique flavors in marinades, broths, and sauces. Pluck some tea from your pantry and indulge in the flavors of Green Tea Sorbet with Candied Ginger and Toasted Walnuts, Black Tea Chicken, Moroccan Mint Tea, or *Masala Chai.*

Grilled Chicken with Walnut and Pomegranate Sauce

The ancient custom of combining meat with fruit is common in Middle Eastern food. This is a lighter version of a classic Iranian stew called *koresh fesenjan,* which is traditionally made with roast duck. Tender grilled chicken breast is served with a sauce of ground walnuts and tangy pomegranate syrup. Garnish with fresh parsley as well as pomegranate seeds if the fruit is in season. Serve with wilted greens and a steaming bowl of whole grains.

Yield: 6 servings
Preparation time: 30 minutes

Walnut and Pomegranate Sauce:
1 tablespoon olive oil
1 cup finely chopped yellow onion
½ teaspoon saffron or turmeric
¼ teaspoon cinnamon
¼ teaspoon nutmeg
¼ teaspoon pepper
2 cups fat-free chicken or vegetable broth
½ cup chopped walnuts

¼ cup pomegranate syrup (see Note below)
1 tablespoon sorghum syrup or dark honey
Salt and pepper to taste

Grilled Chicken:
6 (3-ounce) boneless, skinless chicken breast halves
1 tablespoon olive oil
Salt and pepper to taste

Garnish:
¼ cup chopped fresh Italian parsley, without stems
½ cup pomegranate seeds (optional and if fruit is in season)

Prepare sauce: Heat oil in a large sauté pan over medium heat. Add the onion and cook until softened and light golden brown, about 8 minutes. Add the spices and cook until fragrant, about 1 minute.

Add 1½ cups of the broth and bring to a boil. Reduce heat to low and simmer 5 minutes. Remove from heat.

Place walnuts in the bowl of a food processor and process until very finely ground. Add remaining ½ cup chicken broth, the pomegranate syrup, and the sorghum syrup; process until sauce is creamy and smooth. Carefully add the hot broth and onion mixture; process until smooth.

Return sauce to sauté pan and bring to a boil. Reduce heat and simmer until mixture has the consistency of thick cream, about 3 minutes. Season with salt and pepper. Keep warm.

Prepare chicken: Preheat charcoal grill. Brush chicken lightly with olive oil. Arrange chicken on a rack set about 6 inches over glowing coals. Grill about 4 minutes on each side or until just cooked through. (Alternatively, chicken may be grilled on a hot, ridged grill pan over medium-high heat.) Season with salt and pepper.

Serve each chicken breast with 2 tablespoons sauce and garnish with chopped parsley and pomegranate seeds (if available). Pass extra sauce separately.

NOTE: Pomegranate syrup (also called pomegranate molasses or pomegranate concentrate) can be found in Middle Eastern markets and in the ethnic section of some supermarkets. It is made from the reduced juice of fresh pomegranates. It is a tangy and flavorful addition to salad dressings, marinades, and sauces.

Pomegranate Factoid: The ancient pomegranate has more historical symbolism than most fruit. Its average of 800 seeds may explain its association to fertility rituals and Aphrodite. Its nutritional attributes don't guarantee procreation, but it's ranked in the top echelon with green tea and red wine in terms of antioxidant brawn.

Nutrient Analysis: per serving

CALORIES: 226   PROTEIN: 25 grams   CARBS.: 12 grams   TOTAL FAT: 8 grams   SAT. FAT: 1 gram

POLY. FAT: 3 grams   MONO. FAT: 4 grams   CHOLES.: 58 mgs   FIBER: 1 gram   SODIUM: 94 mgs

Black Tea Chicken with Ginger and Mint

The intermingling of Asian flavors in this dusky tea-based marinade yields a light and sophisticated approach to an easy meal. Serve with whole grains, mushrooms, and braised cabbage.

YIELD: 4 SERVINGS

PREPARATION TIME: 30 MINUTES PLUS 2 HOURS FOR MARINATING

2 cups fat-free chicken or vegetable broth
¼ cup black tea leaves (such as Earl Grey or Darjeeling)
1 tablespoon coarsely chopped fresh mint leaves, without stems
1 tablespoon peeled, chopped fresh ginger
1 tablespoon grated orange peel
1 teaspoon chopped garlic

4 (4-ounce) boneless, skinless chicken breast halves
Salt and pepper to taste
1 tablespoon olive oil

Bring broth to a boil in a 1-quart saucepan over medium heat. Add tea leaves, remove from heat, and allow to infuse 3 minutes. Strain liquid through a fine-meshed sieve into a medium stainless-steel mixing bowl.

Add mint, ginger, orange peel, and garlic to hot tea; allow to cool completely. Add chicken to marinade and refrigerate for a minimum of 2 hours and preferably overnight.

Remove chicken from marinade and pat dry. Season chicken with salt and pepper. Heat oil in a large nonstick sauté pan over medium heat. Add chicken and sauté for 4 minutes, then turn chicken over. Cook until just cooked through, about 4 minutes. Serve immediately.

Mint Factoid: All of the herbs in the mint family, especially oregano and rosemary, are remarkably high in antioxidants.

Nutrient Analysis: per serving

CALORIES: 172   PROTEIN: 29 grams   CARBS.: 1 gram   TOTAL FAT: 5 grams   SAT. FAT: 1 gram
POLY. FAT: 1 gram   MONO. FAT: 3 grams   CHOLES.: 66 mgs   FIBER: 0 gram   SODIUM: 160 mgs

Caponata (Roasted Eggplant Salad)

This Sicilian side dish can be served as a salad or a relish, and it is perfect fare for a picnic. It tastes even better if its flavors have a chance to marry for a day or so.

YIELD: 3 CUPS; 6 (½-CUP) SERVINGS

PREPARATION TIME: 45 MINUTES

6 cups ½-inch dice unpeeled eggplant (about 1½ pounds)
½ medium red onion, halved lengthwise

1 tablespoon extra-virgin olive oil
1 finely chopped medium stalk celery
½ cup pitted, sliced green olives
3 tablespoons tiny nonpareil capers
¼ cup chopped sun-dried tomatoes
1 cup tomato sauce
¼ cup red wine vinegar or balsamic vinegar
1 tablespoon sorghum syrup or dark honey
1 tablespoon unsweetened natural cocoa powder
Salt and pepper to taste
1 tablespoon chopped fresh Italian parsley, without stems
1 tablespoon chopped fresh basil leaves
2 tablespoons toasted pine nuts (see Note below)

Position a rack in lower third of oven. Preheat oven to 450 degrees Fahrenheit. Lightly coat a 15 x 10-inch baking sheet with olive oil spray.

Spread the eggplant in a single layer on the baking sheet; lightly spray with olive oil spray. Roast the eggplant for 8 minutes; turn and roast another 8 minutes, or until softened. Set aside to cool.

Slice off top and bottom ends of onion halves. Place onion on a cutting board with the trimmed bottom end facing you, and while holding the knife at a 45-degree angle, make thin vertical slices.

Heat olive oil in a large sauté pan over medium heat. Add onion and sauté until it just begins to color, about 4 minutes. Stir in celery and cook 1 minute. Stir in the olives, capers, sun-dried tomatoes, tomato sauce, vinegar, sorghum syrup, and cocoa powder; simmer 5 minutes.

Stir in eggplant and simmer 10 minutes. Season with salt and pepper. Stir in herbs and pine nuts. Caponata can be served hot, cold, or at room temperature.

NOTE: To toast pine nuts, spread nuts on an ungreased baking pan. Bake in a preheated 350-degree Fahrenheit oven about 6 minutes, stirring occasionally, or until golden brown.

Cocoa Factoids: Of all chocolate products, cocoa powder has the highest concentration of antioxidant polyphenols. It contains nearly twice the amount found in dark chocolate bars and four times that in milk chocolate bars without all of the added fat and sugar.

Roasted cocoa beans yield chocolate liquor. The amount of liquor in the chocolate end product is the determinant of flavonoid content. Dark chocolates are richest in liquor (and flavonoids) whereas semisweet and milk chocolates have less. White chocolate has none.

Nutrient Analysis: per ½-cup serving

CALORIES: 113   PROTEIN: 3 grams   CARBS.: 15 grams   TOTAL FAT: 6 grams   SAT. FAT: 1 gram
POLY. FAT: 3 grams   MONO. FAT: 1 gram   CHOLES.: 0 mg   FIBER: 3 grams (Sol. 1 gram)
SODIUM: 429 mgs

Nutty Tomato Pesto

Dress up a sandwich or spike a sauce with this easy recipe. Experiment with different nuts, try roasted peppers instead of tomatoes, or use arugula if basil is out of season.

YIELD: 1⅛ CUPS; 18 (1-TABLESPOON) SERVINGS
PREPARATION TIME: 15 MINUTES

1 packed cup fresh basil leaves, without stems
2 tablespoons minced garlic
2 tablespoons chopped sun-dried tomatoes
¾ cup toasted walnuts or almonds (see Note, pages 31 and 133)
¼ teaspoon salt (optional)
⅛ teaspoon ground pepper
½ cup extra-virgin olive oil
⅓ cup grated Romano cheese

Place basil, garlic, tomatoes, walnuts, salt (if using), and pepper in the bowl of a food processor or in a blender jar. Pulse the motor until the walnuts are finely chopped. With the motor running, add oil in a stream. Pulse to blend. Stop and scrape down the sides two or three times to purée evenly. Add the cheese and process 10 to 15 seconds. Do not over-process; the pesto should have some texture.

Transfer to a bowl, cover surface with plastic wrap, and refrigerate up to 1 week.

Nut Factoid: Because nuts are high in fat, they become rancid if exposed to light and heat. For optimal shelf life, keep nuts stored in airtight containers in the freezer.

Nutrient Analysis: per 1-tablespoon serving

CALORIES: 94 PROTEIN: 2 grams CARBS.: 1 gram TOTAL FAT: 9 grams SAT. FAT: 1 gram POLY. FAT: 2 grams MONO. FAT: 5 grams CHOLES.: 2 mgs FIBER: 1 gram SODIUM: 30 mgs

Green Tea Sorbet with Candied Ginger and Toasted Walnuts

Maccha is a green Japanese tea that is delicately processed to retain its rich jade color. The leaves are steamed, dried, and then pulverized into a very fine powder. *Maccha* is an exclusive tea used for formal tea ceremonies in Japan. It is expensive, but a little bit goes a long way. There may be extra effort involved in procuring your *maccha,* but this sorbet makes it worthwhile.

YIELD: 2½ CUPS; 5 (½-CUP) SERVINGS

PREPARATION TIME: 1 HOUR

2 cups vanilla soymilk
2 tablespoons sorghum syrup or dark honey
1½ teaspoons maccha *powder (see Note, page 214)*

2 large egg whites
1 large egg
½ teaspoon pure vanilla extract
¼ cup finely chopped crystallized ginger (see Note, page 119)
3 tablespoons chopped toasted walnuts (see Note, page 31)

Pour soymilk into a 1-quart saucepan over medium heat; warm until it just reaches the boiling point. Remove from heat. Whisk in sorghum syrup and *maccha* powder.

Whisk egg whites and egg in the top of a double boiler until blended. Gradually whisk hot soymilk mixture into the eggs. Place the mixture over simmering water and cook over low heat, whisking gently, until mixture just comes to a boil. The mixture will thicken slightly. Strain mixture into medium mixing bowl; add vanilla and ginger. Let cool 20 minutes. Cover and refrigerate until cold.

Freeze in an ice-cream machine according to the manufacturer's instructions. Stir in walnuts just before removing from machine. If you do not have an ice-cream maker, place the "custard" mixture in the freezer and partially freeze. Remove it from the freezer a few times during the freezing process and mix well with a hand mixer or pulse with a food processor to break up ice crystals. Stir in walnuts at the end and freeze to desired consistency.

NOTE: *Maccha* is a high-quality, bright-green tea powder used in tea ceremonies and in cooking. *Maccha* powder is available in specialty food and tea shops. See Shopping Sources (pages 235–237).

Green Tea Factoid: Green tea leaves are steamed, which prevents their key antioxidant compound, epigallocatechin gallate (EGCG), from oxidizing.

Nutrient Analysis: per ½-cup serving

CALORIES: 153   PROTEIN: 7 grams   CARBS.: 20 grams   TOTAL FAT: 5 grams   SAT. FAT: 1 gram
POLY. FAT: 2 grams   MONO. FAT: 1 gram   CHOLES.: 43 mgs   FIBER: 0 gram   SODIUM: 94 mgs

Banana-Caramel "Ice Cream" with Toasted Walnuts

One day I spent so much time preparing for an elaborate dinner party that I forgot about dessert. Just before my guests arrived, I eyed a basket of ripe bananas on the counter and voilà! This was the hands-down hit of the meal. Sorghum syrup gives a caramel flavor to this frosty treat, and toasting enhances the flavor of omega-3-rich walnuts.

YIELD: 1 QUART; 6 (¾-CUP) SERVINGS
PREPARATION TIME: ABOUT 1 HOUR

2 cups unflavored soymilk
⅓ to ½ cup sorghum syrup, depending on ripeness of bananas
2 egg whites
1 large egg
2 teaspoons pure vanilla extract
4 very ripe medium bananas (about 1¼ pounds before peeling), peeled
*   and cut into large chunks*
2 tablespoons fresh lime juice
⅓ cup chopped, toasted walnuts (see Note, page 31)

Pour soymilk into a 1-quart saucepan over medium heat; warm until it just reaches the boiling point. Remove from heat. Whisk in sorghum syrup.

Whisk egg whites and egg in the top of a double boiler until blended. Gradually whisk hot soymilk mixture into the eggs. Place the mixture over simmering water and cook over low heat, whisking gently, until mixture just comes to a boil and thickens slightly. Strain mixture into medium mixing bowl; add vanilla. Let cool 20 minutes.

Meanwhile, place bananas and lime juice in the bowl of a food processor or blender. Process or blend to a smooth purée. Add banana purée to milk mixture. Cover and refrigerate until cold.

Freeze in an ice-cream machine according to the manufacturer's instructions. Stir in walnuts just before removing from machine. If you do not have an ice-cream maker, place the "custard" mixture in the freezer and partially freeze. Remove it from the freezer a few times during the freezing process and mix well with a hand mixer or pulse with a food processor to break up ice crystals. Stir in walnuts at the end and freeze to desired consistency.

Walnut Factoid: A key factor in the stellar nutritional profile of walnuts is their high-quality protein, attributable to their favorable pattern of important amino acids. One-third cup of walnuts contains the same amount of protein as 1 ounce of meat.

Nutrient Analysis: per ¾-cup serving
CALORIES: 208 PROTEIN: 6 grams CARBS.: 34 grams TOTAL FAT: 6 grams SAT. FAT: 1 gram
POLY. FAT: 4 grams MONO. FAT: 1 gram CHOLES.: 35 mgs FIBER: 4 grams SODIUM: 44 mgs

Mexican Hot Chocolate

For centuries, Mexicans have combined chocolate with spices in their rich savory *mole* dishes. Their traditional hot chocolate drink is reminiscent of this distinctive combination. This blending of antioxidant-rich cocoa powder with cinnamon and cloves yields a soothing beverage that is rich and exotic. And if you're a chocolate purist, you can omit the spices in this recipe.

YIELD: 1½ QUARTS; 6 (1-CUP) SERVINGS
PREPARATION TIME: 10 MINUTES

¼ cup unsweetened natural cocoa powder
6 cups vanilla soymilk
½ cup sorghum syrup or dark honey
1 (3-inch) cinnamon stick, broken in half, or ¼ teaspoon ground cinnamon

10 whole cloves or ⅛ teaspoon ground
1 teaspoon pure vanilla extract

Place cocoa powder in a 2-quart saucepan. Add enough of the soymilk, about ½ cup, to make a smooth paste. Stir well to remove all lumps. Gradually whisk in remaining soymilk and sorghum syrup. Add spices to pan and place over medium-high heat.

Bring hot chocolate just to a simmer; do not boil. Reduce heat to very low and allow to steep 5 minutes. Stir in vanilla. Strain into 6 mugs.

Cocoa Factoid: The high starch content of unsweetened cocoa powder makes it difficult to dissolve in liquid. To prevent lumps from forming, use cold liquid, which can help separate the starch particles.

Nutrient Analysis: per 1-cup serving

CALORIES: 132   PROTEIN: 8 grams   CARBS.: 17 grams   TOTAL FAT: 5 grams   SAT. FAT: 1 gram
POLY. FAT: 1 gram   MONO. FAT: 2 grams   CHOLES.: 0 mg   FIBER: 3 grams   SODIUM: 31 mgs

Masala Chai

The fragrance of *Masala Chai* is as intoxicating as its complex flavor. Traditionally prepared by steeping spices in hot water and milk before adding black tea, this rendition uses green tea instead. It is soothing, restorative, and takes just minutes to prepare.

YIELD: 6 CUPS; 6 (1-CUP) SERVINGS
PREPARATION TIME: 10 MINUTES

4 cups water
6 (¼-inch-thick) slices peeled fresh ginger
½ teaspoon ground cardamom

1 (3-inch) cinnamon stick
6 whole cloves
6 green tea bags
2 cups vanilla soymilk
3 tablespoons sorghum syrup or dark honey

Combine water, ginger, cardamom, cinnamon, and cloves in a small saucepan over medium heat. Bring to a boil, then reduce the heat and simmer about 3 minutes. Remove from heat.

Steep tea bags in the spice mixture for 5 minutes. Strain into a container and store up to 1 week in the refrigerator.

To serve, combine the tea concentrate with the soymilk in a small saucepan. Simmer over low heat but do not boil. Whisk in sorghum syrup. (To prepare a single cup, mix ⅔ cup hot tea concentrate with ⅓ cup hot soymilk. Sweeten with ½ tablespoon sorghum syrup.)

Green Tea Factoid: Doubling the tea's infusion time from 3 to 6 minutes may double the caffeine content, too.

Nutrient Analysis: per ½-cup serving

CALORIES: 80   PROTEIN: 2 grams   CARBS.: 15 grams   TOTAL FAT: 1 gram   SAT. FAT: 0 gram

POLY. FAT: 0 gram   MONO. FAT: 1 gram   CHOLES.: 0 mg   FIBER: 0 gram   SODIUM: 47 mgs

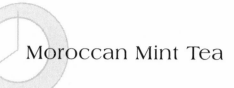

Moroccan Mint Tea

Hot mint tea is served throughout the day in Morocco. It's also delicious iced.

YIELD: 4 CUPS; 4 (1-CUP) SERVINGS
PREPARATION TIME: 10 MINUTES

2 tablespoons loose-leaf green tea or 3 green tea bags
¾ cup lightly packed fresh mint leaves
1 teaspoon grated lemon peel
4 cups boiling water
Sorghum syrup or dark honey (optional)

Place tea, mint leaves, and lemon peel in a pot or small saucepan. Add boiling water, cover, and steep 8 minutes.

Using a strainer, pour tea into small cups or heatproof glasses. Sweeten with sorghum syrup if desired.

Tea Factoid: Green tea is one of the most ancient medicinal agents. One phytochemical in green tea is a catechin called (-)epigallocatechin-3-gallate. It is believed that this compound may beneficially affect certain hormonally modulated activities, such as baldness and acne.

Nutrient Analysis: per 1-cup serving

CALORIES: 1 PROTEIN: 0 gram CARBS.: 0 gram TOTAL FAT: 0 gram SAT. FAT: 0 gram

POLY. FAT: 0 gram MONO. FAT: 0 gram CHOLES: 0 mg FIBER: 0 gram SODIUM: 4 mgs

Selected References

FOREWORD

AARP poll reported in *Time,* 7 June 1999. World Health Organization's Aging and Life Course Division, data from the WHO's Web site: http://www.who.int/hpr/ageing/index.htm.

CHAPTER 1: HOW TO DEFY AGING BY EATING THE FOODS YOU LOVE

Druge, W., "Free Radicals in the Physiological Control of Cell Function." *Physiology Review* 82, 1(2002): 47–95.

Facchini, F. S., et al., "Insulin Resistance as a Predictor of Age-Related Diseases." *Journal of Clinical Endocrinology and Metabolism* 86, 8(August 2001): 3574–3578.

Harman, D., "Free Radical Theory of Aging." *Journal of Gerontology* 11(1956): 298–300.

Martínez-Tomé, M., and A. M. Jiménez, "Antioxidant Properties of Mediterranean Spices Compared with Common Food Additives." *Journal of Food Protection* 64, 9(September 2001): 1412–1419.

Perricone, Nicholas, M.D., F.A.C.N. *The Wrinkle Cure.* New York: Warner Books, 2001.

CHAPTER 2: UNPARALLELED PLUMS AND BERRIES

"Berry Interesting Facts: FAQs." (n.d.) Retrieved July 18, 2001, from the California Strawberry Commission's Web site: http://www.calstrawberry.com/facts/faq.asp.

"Cultivate a Taste for the Blues: Blueberries Up Close and Personal." (n.d.). Retrieved August 23, 2001, from the North American Blueberry Council Web site: http://www.blueberry.org.

"Evaluation of Ellagic Acid Content of Ohio Berries-Final Report: Ohio State University Extension

Information." (n.d.). Retrieved July 18, 2001, from Ohio State University Extension, Midwest Small Fruit and Grape Net Web site: http://www.ag.ohio-staeedu/~sfgnet/eacid_final.html.

Prior, R. L. "Antioxidant Capacity and Health Benefits of Fruits and Vegetables: Blueberries, the Leader of the Pack." (n.d.). Retrieved August 23, 2001, from the North American Blueberry Council Web site: http://www.blueberry.org/tuft's/html.

Prior, R. L., et al., "Antioxidant Capacity as Influenced by Total Phenolic and Anthocyanin Content, Maturity and Variety of Vaccinium Species." *Journal of Agriculture and Food Chemistry* 46(1998): 2686–2693.

"Sweet Sustenance: Strawberry Kitchen Hints." (n.d.). Retrieved July 17, 2001, from the Original Strawberry Facts Page: http://www.jamm.com/strawberry/sustenance.html.

CHAPTER 3: SUPREME CITRUS AND GRAPES

Bok, S. H., et al., "Plasma and Hepatic Cholesterol and Hepatic Activities of 3-Hydroxy-3-Methyl-Glutaryl-CoA Reductase and Acyl CoA: Cholesterol Transferase Are Lower in Rats Fed Citrus Peel Extract or a Mixture of Citrus Bioflavonoids." *Journal of Nutrition* 129, 6(June 1999): 1182–1185.

Calabrese, V., et al., "Biochemical Studies on a Novel Antioxidant from Lemon Oil and Its Biotechnological Application in Cosmetic Dermatology." *Drugs Under Experimental and Clinical Research* 25, 5(1999): 219–225.

Corder, R., et al., "Endothelin-1 Synthesis Reduced by Red Wine." *Nature* 414(2001): 863–864.

Freedman, J. E., et al., "Select Flavonoids and Whole Grape Juice from Purple Grapes Inhibit Platelet Function and Enhance Nitric Oxide Release." *Circulation* 103(2001): 279–298.

Fuhrman, B., et al., "White Wine with Red-Wine-like Properties: Increased Extraction of Grape Skin Polyphenols Improves the Antioxidant Capacity of Derived White Wine." *Journal of Agriculture and Food Chemistry* 49, 7(2001): 3164–3168.

Kurowska, E. M., et al., "HDL-Cholesterol-Raising Effect of Orange Juice in Subjects with Hypercholesterolemia." *American Journal of Clinical Nutrition* 72, 5(November 2000): 1095–1100.

Liu, R. H., et al., "Antioxidant and Antiproliferative Activities of Grapes." (n.d.). Retrieved September 11, 2001, from http://ift.confex.com/ift/2001/techprogram/paper_8142.html.

Mangels, A. R., et al., "Carotenoid Content of Fruits and Vegetables: An Evaluation of Analytic Data." *Journal of the American Dietetics Association* 93, 3(March 1993): 284–296.

Seddon, J. M., et al., "Dietary Carotenoids, Vitamins A, C, and E, and Advanced Age-Related Macular Degeneration." *Journal of the American Medical Association* 272, 18(November 9, 1994): 1413–1420.

Stein, J. H., et al., "Purple Grape Juice Improves Endothelial Function and Reduces the Susceptibility of LDL Cholesterol to Oxidation in Patients with Coronary Artery Disease." *Circulation* 100(1999): 1050–1055.

CHAPTER 4: TIME-HONORED TOMATOES

Djuric, Z., and L. C. Powell, "Antioxidant Capacity of Lycopene-Containing Foods." *International Journal of Food Science and Nutrition* 52, 2(March 2001): 143–149.

Giovannucci, E., et al., "Intake of Carotenoids and Retinol in Relation to Risk of Prostate Cancer." *Journal of the National Cancer Institute* 87, 23(December 6, 1995): 1767–1776.

Heber, D., Q. Y. Lu, and V. L. Go, "Role of Tomatoes, Tomato Products and Lycopene in Cancer Prevention." *Advances in Experimental and Medical Biology* 492(2001): 29–37.

Lu, Q. Y., et al., "Inverse Associations between Plasma Lycopene and Other Carotenoids and Prostate Cancer." *Cancer Epidemiology, Biomarkers, and Prevention* 10, 7(July 2001): 749–756.

Ribaya-Mercado, J. D., et al., "Skin Lycopene Is Destroyed Preferentially over Beta-Carotene During Ultraviolet Irradiation in Humans." *Journal of Nutrition* 125, 7(1995): 1854–1859.

CHAPTER 5: AROMATIC TRIO: GINGER, ONIONS, AND GARLIC

Amagase, H., et al., "Intake of Garlic and Its Bioactive Components." *Journal of Nutrition* 131(2001): 955S–962S.

Borchers, A. T., et al., "Inflammation and Native American Medicine: The Role of Botanicals 1, 2, 3." *American Journal of Clinical Nutrition* 72, 2(August 2000): 339–347.

Craig, W. J., "Health-Promoting Properties of Common Herbs." *American Journal of Clinical Nutrition* 70(Suppl.) (1999): 491S–499S.

Fleischauer, A. T., C. Poole, and L. Arab, "Garlic Consumption and Cancer Prevention: Meta-Analyses of Colorectal and Stomach Cancers 1, 2, 3." *American Journal of Clinical Nutrition* 72, 4(October 2000): 1047–1052.

Hertog, M. G., et al., "Dietary Antioxidant Flavonoids and Risk of Coronary Heart Disease: The Zutphen Elderly Study." *Lancet* 342, 8878(October 23, 1993): 1007–1011.

Howard, B., and D. Kritchevsky, "Phytochemicals and Cardiovascular Disease." *Circulation* 95 (1997): 2591–2593.

Martínez-Tomé, M., and A. M. Jiménez, "Antioxidant Properties of Mediterranean Spices Compared with Common Food Additives." *Journal of Food Protection* 64, 9(September 2001): 1412–1419.

Robert, V., et al., "Effects of the Garlic Compound Diallyl Disulfide on the Metabolism, Adherence and Cell Cycle of HT-29 Colon Carcinoma Cells: Evidence of Sensitive and Resistant Sub-Populations." *Carcinogenesis* 22, 8(August 2001): 1155–1161.

Tyler, V., "Spotlight on Ginger." *Prevention* 50, 2(February 1998): 82–85.

CHAPTER 6: GLORIOUS GREENS

Beecher, C. W., "Cancer Preventive Properties of Varieties of *Brassica oleracea:* A Review." *American Journal of Clinical Nutrition* 59(1994): 1166S–1170S.

Cao, G., et al., "Antioxidant Capacity of Tea and Common Vegetables." *Journal of Agriculture and Food Chemistry* 44(1996): 3426–3431.

Duester, K., "Avocado Fruit Is a Rich Source of Beta-Sitosterol." *Journal of the American Dietetics Association* 101(2001): 404–405.

Goda, Y., et al., "Constituents in Watercress: Inhibitors of Histamine Release from RBL-2H3 Cells Induced by Antigen Stimulation." *Biological and Pharmaceutical Bulletin* 22, 12(December 1999): 1319–1326.

Kurilich, A. C., et al., "Carotene, Tocopherol, and Ascorbate Contents of Subspecies of *Brassica oleracea*." *Journal of Agriculture and Food Chemistry* 47, 4(1999): 1576–1581.

McBride, J., "Can Foods Forestall Aging?" *Agricultural Research* 47, 2(February 1999): 15–17.

Prince, P., and G. Waldon. Press release: "Presidential Candidates Duck the Crucial Broccoli Question: America Wants to Know: 'Will the Cancer Fighting Benefits of Broccoli Find a Place at the Table?'" (September 20, 2000). Retrieved September 12, 2001, from the American Institute for Cancer Research Web site: http://www.aicr.org/r092000.html.

Sawa, T., et al., "Alkylperoxyl Radical-Scavenging Activity of Various Flavonoids and Other Phenolic Compounds: Implications for the Anti-Tumor-Promoter Effect of Vegetables." *Journal of Agriculture and Food Chemistry* 47, 2(February 1999): 397–402.

Van Poppel, G., et al., "Brassica Vegetables and Cancer Prevention: Epidemiology and Mechanisms." *Advances in Experimental and Medical Biology* 472(1999): 159–168.

CHAPTER 7: SENSATIONAL SOY

Burow, M. E., et al., "Phytochemical Glyceollins, Isolated from Soy, Mediate Antihormonal Effects Through Estrogen Receptor Alpha and Beta." *Journal of Clinical Endocrinology and Metabolism* 86(2001): 1750–1758.

Ingram, D., et al., "Case-Control Study of Phytoestrogens and Breast Cancer." *Lancet* 350(1997): 990–994.

Lu, L. J., et al., "Phytoestrogens and Healthy Aging: Gaps in Knowledge. A Workshop Report." *Menopause* 3(2001): 157–170.

Messina, M. J., "Legumes and Soybeans: Overview of Their Nutritional Properties and Health Effects." *American Journal of Clinical Nutrition* 70(Suppl.) (1999): 439S–450S.

Scheiber, M. D., et al., "Dietary Inclusion of Whole Soy Foods Results in Significant Reductions in Clinical Risk Factors for Osteoporosis and Cardiovascular Disease in Normal Postmenopausal Women." *Menopause* 8(2001): 384–392.

Sirtori, C. R., and M. R. Lovati, "Soy Proteins and Cardiovascular Disease." *Current Atherosclerosis Reports* 3(2001): 47–53.

Slavin, J. L., M. C. Martini, and D. R. Jacobs Jr., "Plausible Mechanisms for the Protectiveness of Whole Grains." *American Journal of Clinical Nutrition* 70(Suppl.) (1999): 459S–463S.

Tikkanen, M. J., and H. Aldercreutz, "Dietary Soy-Derived Isoflavone Phytoestrogens: Could They Have a Role in Coronary Heart Disease Prevention?" *Biochemical Pharmacology* 60(2000): 1–5.

Visioli, F., L. Borsanni, and C. Galli, "Diet and Prevention of Heart Disease: The Potential Role of Phytochemicals." *Cardiovascular Research* 47(2000): 419–425.

CHAPTER 8: COLORFUL CARROTS, BEETS, BELL PEPPERS, PUMPKINS, SWEET POTATOES, AND MANGOES

Fortin, F. (ed.), *The Visual Food Encyclopedia: The Definitive Practical Guide to Food and Cooking.* New York: Macmillan, 1996. P. 61.

Hands, E. S., *Food Finder: Vitamin and Mineral Source Guide.* 3d ed. Salem, OR: ESHA Research, 1995.

Jonsson, L., "Thermal Degradation of Carotenes and Influence on Their Physiological Functions." *Advances in Experimental and Medical Biology* 289(1991): 75–82.

Karaman, S., et al., "Antibacterial and Antifungal Activity of the Essential Oils of Thymus Revolutus Celak from Turkey." *Journal of Ethnopharmacology* 76, 2(July 2001): 183–186.

Litz, R. E. (ed.), *The Mango: Botany, Production and Uses.* New York: CAB International, 1997.

Rodríguez-Amaya, D. B., "Latin American Food Sources of Carotenoids." *Archives of Latino American Nutrition* 3(Suppl. 1) (September 1999): 74S–84S.

Talcot, S. T., et al., "Antioxidant Changes and Sensory Properties of Carrot Puree Processed with and without Periderm Tissue." *Journal of Agricultural and Food Chemistry* 48(2000): 1315–1321.

University of California Cooperative Extension Tulare County Agriculture and Natural Resources. "Yam or Sweet Potato?" *UCCE News.* (n.d.)

CHAPTER 9: SPLENDID GRAINS AND SEEDS

Asp, N. G., "Resistant Starch—An Update on Its Physiological Effects." *Advances in Experimental and Medical Biology* 427(1997): 201–210.

Cooney, R. V., et al., "AA Effects of Dietary Sesame Seeds on Plasma Tocopherol Levels." *Nutrition and Cancer* 39, 1(2001): 66–71.

Gordon, L. A., et al., "Characteristics of Breads Baked with Sorghum Brans High in Phenolic Compounds." 2001 Sorghum Industry Conference and 22nd Biennial Grain Sorghum Research and Utilization Conference, February 18–20, Nashville, TN, pp. 98–102.

Jacobs, D. R., Jr., et al., "'Is Whole-Grain Intake Associated with Reduced Total and Cause-Specific Death Rates in Older Women?' The Iowa Women's Health Study." *American Journal of Public Health* 89(1999): 322–329.

———, "Whole-Grain Intake May Reduce the Risk of Ischemic Heart Disease Death in Post-Menopausal Women: The Iowa Women's Health Study." *American Journal of Clinical Nutrition* 68(1998): 248–257.

Katz, D. L., et al., "Effects of Oat and Wheat Cereals on Endothelial Responses." *Preventive Medicine* 33, 5(November 2001): 476–484.

Mazur, W., and H. Adlercreutz, "Natural and Anthropogenic Environmental Estrogens: The Scientific Basis for Risk Assessment: Naturally Occurring Estrogens in Food." *Pure and Applied Chemistry* 70, 9(1998): 1759–1776.

Murkovic, M., et al., "Variability of Fatty Acid Content in Pumpkin Seeds (Cucurbita pepol)." *Zeitschrift für Lebensmittel-Untersuchung und-Forschung* 203, 3(1996): 216–219.

Nishizawa, N., et al., "Proso Millet Protein Elevates Plasma Level of High-Density Lipoprotein: A New Food Function of Proso Millet." *Biomedical and Environmental Sciences* 9, 2–3(September 1996): 209–212.

Slavin, J. L., et al., "Plausable Mechanisms for the Protectiveness of Whole Grains." *American Journal of Clinical Nutrition* 70(Suppl.) (1999): 459S–463S.

Wilson, T. A., et al., "Corn Fiber Oil Lowers Plasma Cholesterol Levels and Increases Cholesterol Excretion Greater Than Corn Oil and Similar to Diets Containing Soy Sterols and Soy Stanols in Hamsters." *Journal of Nutritional Biochemistry* 11, 9(September 1, 2000): 443–449.

CHAPTER 10: BOUNTIFUL BEANS AND LEGUMES

Asp, N. G., "Resistant Starch—An Update on Its Physiological Effects." *Advances in Experimental and Medical Biology* 427(1997): 201–210.

Awad, A. N., et al., "Peanuts as a Source of Beta-Sitosterol, a Sterol with Anticancer Properties." *Nutrition and Cancer* 36(2000): 238–241.

Gibson, G. R., and M. B. Roberfroid, "Dietary Modulation of the Human Colonic Microbiota: Introducing the Concept of Prebiotics." *Journal of Nutrition* 125(1995): 1401–1412.

Kushi, L. H., K. A. Meyer, and D. R. Jacobs Jr., "Cereals, Legumes, and Chronic Disease Risk Reduction: Evidence from Epidemiologic Studies." *American Journal of Clinical Nutrition* 70(3 Suppl.) (September 1999): 451S–458S.

"Pea, Chickpea, and Lentil Information." (n.d.). Retrieved August 31, 2001, from the U.S.A. Dry Pea and Lentil Council Web site: http://www.pea-lentil.com/nutrition.html.

Rabey, J. M., et al., "Broad Bean *(Vicia faba)* Consumption and Parkinson's Disease." *Advances in Neurology* 60(1993): 681–684.

Rao, A. V., "Anticarcinogenic Properties of Plant Saponins." Abstract in Second International Symposium on the Role of Soy in Preventing and Treating Chronic Disease, September 1996, Brussels, Belgium.

Rotondo, S., et al., "Effect of Trans-Resveratrol, a Natural Polyphenolic Compound, on Human Polymorphonuclear Leukocyte Function." *British Journal of Pharmacology* 123(1998): 1691–1699.

Salmeron, J., et al., "Dietary Fiber, Glycemic Load, and Risk of NIDDM in Men." *Diabetes Care* 20(1997): 545–550.

Salmeron, J., et al., "Dietary Fiber, Glycemic Load, and Risk of Non-Insulin Dependent Diabetes Mellitus in Women." *Journal of the American Medical Association* 277(1997): 472–477.

CHAPTER 11: FABULOUS FISH AND FLAX

Albert, C. M., "Fish Consumption and Risk of Sudden Cardiac Death." *Journal of the American Medical Association* 279(1998): 23–28.

Caygill, C. P. J., and M. J. Hill, "Fish, N-3 Fatty Acids and Human Colorectal and Breast Cancer Mortality." *European Journal of Cancer Prevention* 4(1995): 329–332.

Connor, W. E., "Importance of N-3 Fatty Acids in Health and Disease." *American Journal of Clinical Nutrition* 71(Suppl.) (2000): 171S–175S.

De Caterina, R., J. K. Liao, and P. Libby, "Fatty Acid Modulation of Endothelial Activation." *American Journal of Clinical Nutrition* 71(Suppl.) (2000): 213S–223S.

James, M. J., R. A. Gibson, and L. G. Cleland, "Dietary Polyunsaturated Fatty Acids and Inflammatory Mediator Production." *American Journal of Clinical Nutrition* 71(Suppl.) (2000): 343S–348S.

Kang, J. X., and A. Leaf, "Antiarrhythmic Effects of Polyunsaturated Fatty Acids." *Circulation* 94(1996): 1774–1780.

Kremer, J. M., "N-3 Fatty Acid Supplements in Rheumatoid Arthritis." *American Journal of Clinical Nutrition* 71(Suppl.) (2000): 349S–351S.

Lloyd-Still, J. D., et al., "Essential Fatty Acid Deficiency and Predisposition to Lung Disease in Cystic Fibrosis." *Acta Paediatr* 85, 12(1996): 1426–1432.

Norrish, A. E., "Prostate Cancer Risk and Consumption of Fish Oils: A Dietary Biomarker-Based Case-Control Study." *British Journal of Cancer* 81(1999): 1238–1242.

Schwartz, J., and S. T. Weiss, "The Relationship of Dietary Fish Intake to Level of Pulmonary Function in the First National Health And Nutrition Survey (NHANES)." *European Respir. Journal* 7(1994): 1821–1824.

Smith, W., P. Mitchell, and S. R. Leeder, "Dietary Fat and Fish Intake and Age-Related Maculopathy." *Archives of Ophthalmology* 118(March 2000): 401–404.

CHAPTER 12: NOBLE NUTS, COCOA, AND TEA

Awad, A. B., and C. S. Fink, "Phytosterols as Anticancer Dietary Components: Evidence and Mechanism of Action." *Journal of Nutrition* 130(2000): 2127–2130.

Belguendouz, L., L. Fremont, and M. T. Gozzelino, "Interaction of Transresveratrol with Plasma Lipoproteins." *Biochemical Pharmacology* 55(1998): 811–816.

Connor, W. E., "The Beneficial Effects of Omega-3 Fatty Acids: Cardiovascular Disease and Neurodevelopment." *Current Opinions in Lipidology* 8(1997): 1–3.

Dreosti, I. E., "Bioactive Ingredients: Antioxidants and Polyphenols in Tea." *Nutrition Reviews* 54(1996): S51–S58.

Hertog, M. G., et al., "Dietary Antioxidant Flavonoids and Risk of Coronary Heart Disease: The Zutphen Elderly Study." *Lancet,* 8878(October 23, 1993): 1007–1011.

Hirano, R., et al., "Antioxidant Effect of Polyphenols in Chocolate on Low-Density Lipoprotein Both in Vitro and Ex Vivo." *Journal of Nutritional Science and Vitaminology* 46(2000): 199–204.

Ishikawa, T., et al., "Effect of Tea Flavonoid Supplementation on the Susceptibility of Low-Density Lipoprotein to Oxidative Modification." *American Journal of Clinical Nutrition* 66(1997): 261–266.

Jang, M., et al., "Cancer Chemopreventive Activity of Resveratrol, a Natural Product Derived from Grapes." *Science* 275(1997): 218–220.

Keen, C. L., "Chocolate: Food as Medicine/Medicine as Food." *Journal of the American College of Nutrition 2001* 20(5 Suppl.) (2001): 436S–439S.

Keli, S. O., et al., "Dietary Flavonoids, Antioxidant Vitamins, and Incidence of Stroke: The Zutphen Study." *Archives of Internal Medicine* 156(1996): 637–642.

Kris-Etherton, P. M., et al., "The Effects of Nuts on Coronary Heart Disease Risk." *Nutrition Reviews* 59 (2001): 103–111.

Leung, L. K., et al., "Theaflavins in Black Tea and Catechins in Green Tea Are Equally Effective Antioxidants." *Journal of Nutrition* 131(2001): 2248–2251.

Liao, S., "The Medicinal Action of Androgens and Green Tea Epigallocatechin Gallate." *Hong Kong Medical Journal* 7, 4(December 2001): 369–374.

Mukhtar, H., et al., "Tea Components: Antimutagenic and Anticarcinogenic Effects." *Preventative Medicine* 21(1992): 351–360.

Rajaram, S., et al., "A Monounsaturated Fatty Acid-Rich Pecan-Enriched Diet Favorably Alters the Serum Lipid Profile of Healthy Men and Women." *Journal of Nutrition* 131(2001): 2275–2279.

Sabate, J., et al., "Effects of Walnuts on Serum Lipid Levels and Blood Pressure in Normal Men." *New England Journal of Medicine* 328(1993): 603–607.

Spiller, G. A., et al., "Nuts and Plasma Lipids: An Almond-Based Diet Lowers LDL-C While Preserving HDL-C." *Journal of the American College of Nutrition* 17(1998): 285–290.

Vinson, J. A., J. Proch, and L. Zubik, "Phenol Antioxidant Quality and Quantity in Foods: Cocoa, Dark Chocolate and Milk Chocolate." *Journal of Agriculture and Food Chemistry* 47(1999): 4821–4824.

On the Web

A4M
www.worldhealth.net
Antiaging medicine site

AMERICAN DIETETIC ASSOCIATION
www.eatright.org
Information on nutrition and food

THE BLONZ GUIDE
http://www.blonz.com
Information on nutrition and food

OLDWAYS PRESERVATION AND EXCHANGE
http://www.oldwayspt.org/

SORGHUM SYRUP INFORMATION
http://www.ca.uky.edu/nssppa/index.html

STOP THE CLOCK! COOKING
www.stoptheclockcooking.com

USDA AGRICULTURAL RESEARCH SERVICE
http://www.ars.usda.gov/is/index.html

USDA PHYTOCHEMICAL LABORATORY
http://www.barc.usda.gov/bhnrc/pl/index.html

Further Reading

Carper, Jean. *Stop Aging Now!: The Ultimate Plan for Staying Young and Reversing the Aging Process.* New York: HarperPerennial, 1996.

Duke, James, Ph.D. *The Green Pharmacy Anti-Aging Prescriptions: Herbs, Foods, and Natural Formulas to Keep You Young.* Emmaus, PA: Rodale, 2001.

Gollman, Barbara, M.S., R.D., and Kim Pierce. *The Phytopia Cookbook.* Phytopia, Inc., 1998.

Heber, David, M.D., Ph.D., and Susan Bowerman, M.S., R.D. *What Color Is Your Diet?* New York: Regan Books, 2001.

Joseph, James A., Daniel A. Nadeau, and Anne Underwood. *The Color Code: A Revolutionary Eating Plan for Optimum Health.* New York: Hyperion, 2002.

Klatz, Ronald, and Robert Goldman. *New Anti-Aging Secrets for Maximum Lifespan.* New York: MDM, Inc., 1999; *Stopping the Clock.* New York: Bantam, 1997; *Stopping the Clock II: Longevity for a New Millennium* (forthcoming).

Mozian, Laurie Deutsch, M.S., R.D. *Foods That Fight Disease.* New York: Avery Books, 2000.

Perricone, Nicholas. *The Perricone Prescription.* New York: HarperCollins, 2002.

Walford, Roy L., M.D. *Beyond the 120 Year Diet: How to Double Your Vital Years.* New York: Four Walls Eight Windows, 2000.

Willcox, Bradley, M.D., and Craig Willcox, Ph.D. *The Okinawa Program.* New York: Clarkson N. Potter, 2001.

Willet, Walter, M.D., P. J. Skerrett, and Edward L. Giovannucci, M.D. *Eat, Drink, and Be Healthy: The Harvard Medical School Guide to Healthy Eating.* New York: Simon & Schuster, 2001.

Shopping Sources

AMERICAN NATURAL AND SPECIALTY
   BRANDS
405 Golfway Drive West
St. Augustine, Florida 32095-8839
Telephone: 800-238-3947
Fax: 904-940-2334
www.ans-natural.com
Chatfield's unsweetened natural cocoa powder

BOB'S RED MILL NATURAL FOODS
5209 SE International Way
Milwaukie, Oregon 97222
Telephone: 800-349-2173
www.bobsredmill.net
Whole-grain flours, sorghum flour, seeds, beans,
   bulk grains

DEAN AND DELUCA
New York, New York
Telephone: 800-999-0306
Chipotle chiles, crystallized ginger, spices, beans,
   lentils, whole grains, pomegranate molasses,
   tahini, sorghum syrup, *maccha* tea, preserved
   lemons

HEINTZMAN FARMS
3138 East 7th Street
Long Beach, California 90804
Telephone: 562-439-7611
www.heintzmanfarms.com
Flaxseed

KALUSTYAN'S
123 Lexington Avenue
New York, New York 10016
Telephone: 212-685-3451
www.kalustyans.com
Spices, teas, beans, grains, chipotle chiles, pomegranate syrup, tahini, preserved lemons

MAASDAM SORGHUM MILLS
6495 East 132nd Street South
Lynnville, Iowa 50153
Telephone: 641-594-4369
E-mail: **sorghum@netins.net**
Sorghum syrup

MAKING TRACKS
P.O. Box 4898
Chatsworth, California 91313-4898
Telephone: 800-488-8898
www.makingtracks.com
E-mail: **Makingtracks@hotmail.com**
Sorghum syrup

PENZEYS SPICES
Telephone: 800-741-7787
Unsweetened natural cocoa powder, spices

SCHARFFEN BERGER CHOCOLATE MAKER,
   INC.
914 Heinz Avenue
Berkeley, California 94710
Telephone: 800-884-5884; 510-981-4050
http://www.scharffenberger.com
Unsweetened natural cocoa powder

SPECIALTEAS, INC.
2 Reynolds Street
Norwalk, Connecticut 06855-1015
Telephone: 888-enjoy-tea (365-6983)
www.specialteas.com
Maccha green tea

SURFAS RESTAURANT SUPPLY AND
   GOURMET FOOD
Culver City, California 90232
Telephone: 310-559-4770
Tahini, spices, unsweetened natural cocoa
   powder, olive oil, pomegranate syrup

TWIN VALLEY MILLS
Rural Route 1, Box 45
Ruskin, Nebraska 68974
Telephone: 402-279-3965
www.twinvalleymills.com
Sorghum flour

LIST OF INDEPENDENT SORGHUM SYRUP
   SOURCES
**www.ca.uky.edu/nssppa/sorghumsources/
   syrup.html**

Updates can be found at
   www.stoptheclockcooking.com

Glossary

Allium compounds are substances found in allium vegetables, which include garlic, onions, leeks, chives and shallots. They are formed and released primarily when the plants are crushed, cut and heated. Examples of allium compounds include ajoenes, diallyl sulfides and allyl methyl trisulfide. This group of phytochemicals has demonstrated many positive health effects, such as decreasing cancer production by detoxifying carcinogens, reducing heart disease by lowering cholesterol and blood pressure and reducing blood clotting.

Allyl methyl trisulfide is a member of the allium family found in onions and garlic, namely garlic oil (see allium compounds definition above). This organosulfur compound has shown promising effects recently in the research areas of cancer and heart disease protection.

Alpha carotene is a member of the class of plant carotenoid pigments and one of the main types of carotene in foods (other examples are [beta]- and [gamma]-carotene). It is a precursor of the fat-soluble Vitamin A, yielding the vitamin once broken down during digestion in the body.

Alpha tocopherol is one of four tocopherols, a group of fat-soluble substances that possess Vitamin E activity and have the key ability to stabilize and protect cell membranes from the damaging effects of oxygen free radicals. They have shown significant antioxidant effects in research. The most important member of the Vitamin E group is alpha-tocopherol, which is the most biologically active Vitamin E compound. Dietary sources include vegetable oils and their products, green leafy vegetables, nuts, seeds and whole grain cereals.

Anthocyanins are one the most abundant types of flavonoids (a major group of phenol phytochemicals) found primarily in fruits, such as berries. These substances are antioxidants and have demonstrated the ability to quench free radicals, decrease unfavorable oxidation of LDL cholesterol and protect against cardiovascular disease.

Antioxidant is a substance that can neutralize oxygen free radicals, the highly reactive and damaging atoms and chemical groups produced by various disease processes and by poisons, radiation and smoking. The body produces its own natural antioxidants, and along with dietary antioxidants, they aid in controlling cell and tissue damage. The most commonly used antioxidants in the diet are Vitamin C, Vitamin E and beta-carotene, as well as a variety of phytochemical substances recently identified in plant foods.

Beta-carotene is a member of a carotenoid class of pigments found in plants. Of all the carotenoids, beta-carotene has the greatest Vitamin A activity, which means it will produce the vitamin in appreciable amounts when it is broken down during human digestion. Aside from being a Vitamin A precursor, beta-carotene functions as an antioxidant to protect the body against disease. Rich food sources include dark green leafy vegetables (spinach, kale) and orange fruits and vegetables (pumpkin, carrots, cantaloupe and sweet potato).

Biochanin A is a substance belonging to the isoflavone group (which also includes genistein and diadzein) found in soy products (see definition of isoflavones below). It has shown potent estrogen-like activity in recent research, namely producing an estrogen blocking effect by tying up estrogen receptors on cells. This plant estrogen activity is being studied with respect to protection against hormone-related cancers, including breast and prostate cancer.

Bioflavonoids is another name for flavonoids (see definition on page 236).

Caffeic acids are substances belonging to the phenolic acid group, which is part of the larger class of phytochemicals, the phenols (see definition on page 240). Found in fruits and vegetables, these acids have demonstrated protection against development of cancer and atherosclerosis. In addition, these phenolic acids are also found in whole grains and are thought to be responsible for the natural antioxidant capacity of grains, especially oats. These substances also influence the sensory quality and stability of food.

Campesterol is a plant substance belonging to the group of phytochemicals called phytosterols, which is similar in structure to cholesterol. It is believed that moderate levels of consumption of campesterol can interfere with cholesterol absorption and result in decreased serum cholesterol levels. Plant sources are beans and oils.

Carcinogens are any substances that cause cancer. Examples include chemicals (i.e., cigarettes), radiation and some viruses.

Carnosol is a phenolic compound found in rosemary that has demonstrated potent antioxidant activity and other beneficial effects, such as preventing unfavorable oxidation of cholesterol and inhibiting cancer.

Carotenoids are yellow, orange and red pigment phytochemicals with antioxidant activity that have exhibited beneficial health effects in scientific studies, such as reducing cancer, cardiovascular disease and macular degeneration. There are over 600 carotenoids identified. Key sources are fruits and vegetables of the colors previously mentioned. Beta-carotene, lycopene, alpha-carotene, lutein, zeaxanthin and betacryptoxanthin are commonly mentioned carotenoid compounds, which have been identified in high concentrations in the human bloodstream.

Catechins are a group of flavonoid compounds that belong to the larger class of phytochemicals called phenols and have demonstrated key antioxidant activity in recent research. Found primarily in green and black tea and wine, catechins have shown promising effects in protecting against heart disease and cancer.

Chalcones are flavonoid compounds (which belong to the larger class of phytochemicals called phenols) found in plants, namely licorice. These substances have been studied recently with respect to possible protection against infection, cancer and heart disease.

Cholesterol is a sterol (fatlike material) made by the liver, which is present in blood and most tissues, especially nervous tissue. Cholesterol functions as a key component of cell membranes and is a precursor of many steroid hormones and bile salts. Aside from being synthesized in the body, cholesterol can be obtained by diet from animal foods such as meats, dairy products and eggs. High dietary intake of saturated fat (also present in foods listed above), more so than dietary cholesterol, is linked to elevated cholesterol in the blood, a condition called hypercholesterolemia.

Coumarins is a class of widely occurring phenolic compounds found in citrus fruits, celery, figs and parsnips. They have demonstrated ability to aid enzymes that fight cancer in recent studies.

Cryptoxanthin is a substance belonging to a class of phytochemicals called the carotenoids (see definition on the previous page) found in citrus and tropical fruits, especially mango, tangerines, oranges and papaya. This plant pigment can be converted to Vitamin A in the body and has demonstrated significant antioxidant activity in research.

Curcumin is a phenolic compound responsible for the yellow color in turmeric and mustard spices. It is also found in ginger. This phytochemical has demonstrated promising anticancer, anti-inflammatory and antioxidant effects.

Cynarin is a phytochemical found in artichoke plants and is believed to lower elevated blood cholesterol. Unlike cholesterol-lowering drugs that can have toxic effects on the liver, cynarin is thought to *improve* liver function.

Dehydroepiandrosterone (DHEA) is a hormone that converts to androgen or estrogen forms and produces beneficial effects believed to protect against coronary artery disease, osteoporosis and possibly weight gain. The aging process is associated with progressive declines in the levels of many hormones including DHEA.

Diadzein is one of the most well-researched isoflavones (a group of flavonoid compounds belonging to the larger class of phytochemicals called phenols—see definition on page 240). It is one of the primary isoflavones in soybeans, and thus soy foods are the richest dietary source of diadzein. Health benefits linked to diadzein and other isoflavones include protection against certain types of cancers, heart disease and osteoporosis.

Disulfides are allium compounds that are found primarily in garlic and are released when it is heated. Research has suggested that these organosulfur compounds may have an anticancer role. They are suspected of being the active ingredient in garlic, which lowers cholesterol and triglycerides (see Allium compounds definition on page 233).

Dithiolthiones are one type of organosulfide (see definition on page 239) that are found primarily in cruciferous vegetables and have been linked to beneficial health effects, namely cancer protection. Research suggests that these substances may aid enzymes that help detoxify carcinogens.

Ellagic acid is a substance belonging to the phenolic acid group, which is part of the larger class of phytochemicals—the phenols (see definition on page 240). Rich sources include fruits such as strawberries, cranberries and blackberries, as well as nuts, such as walnuts. Ellagic acid has been studied with respect to its role in protecting against cancer and heart disease. This substance also influences the sensory quality and stability of food.

Ferulic acid is a substance belonging to the phenolic acid group, which is part of the larger class of phytochemicals—the phenols (see definition on page 240). Found in fruits and vegetables, these acids have demonstrated protection against development of cancer and atherosclerosis. In addition, these phenolic acids are also found in whole grains and are thought to be responsible for their natural antioxidant capacity, namely in oats. This plant substance also influences the sensory quality and stability of food.

Fiber is a material found in plant food, such as nonstarch polysaccharides (cellulose, hemicelluloses, pectins, gums, mucilages) and lignins. It is resistant to human digestion. Its key functions include promoting regularity, lowering cholesterol and blood glucose levels, as well as increasing satiety for weight control. Foods high in fiber are whole grains, legumes, fruits and vegetables.

Flavanones are a member of the flavonoid class of phenol phytochemicals (see definition below). Key sources include citrus fruits.

Flavonoids, also known as bioflavonoids, are a key group of compounds belonging to the phenol class of phytochemicals and one of the most potent types of plant antioxidant compounds. Flavonoids are the most widely researched of all the phenols. Their many potential effects include defending cells against carcinogens, decreasing the unfavorable oxidation of LDL cholesterol and preventing blood clotting. Major flavonoid subclasses include flavonols, flavanones, catechins anthocyanins, isoflavones, dihydroflavonols and chalcones. Sources of flavonoids are widely available in plant food such as fruits, vegetables, legumes, nuts and teas.

Flavonols are a member of the flavonoid class of phenol phytochemicals (see definition on page 240). Key sources include fruits, vegetables and tea.

Folic acid is a water-soluble B vitamin that is a part of the enzyme machinery involved in making DNA and is therefore key to new cell formation. Significant food sources include green leafy vegetables, legumes and seeds.

Free radical is a very reactive, unstable molecule, formed during normal human metabolism, that is missing an electron in one of its own atoms. A free radical will steal an electron from another molecule, transforming the second molecule into a free radical (as the second one now lacks an electron). This can start a chain reaction in the body that ultimately leads to cell damage if the free radical is not stopped by pairing with a molecule that has a single electron to give. Antioxidants can also break the chain reaction and inhibit free radicals.

Functional food is a food consumed for specified health purposes, because of its high content of one or more nutrients or non-nutrient substances that may confer health benefits. In 1994, the Food and Nutrition Board of the American Institute of Medicine defined "functional food" as "any modified food or food ingredient that may provide a health benefit beyond the traditional nutrients it contains." Examples of functional foods can be macronutrients (i.e., omega-fatty acid-enriched products), larger doses of added micronutrients (i.e., vitamin and mineral contents greater than Recommended Daily Intake) or even substances with no actual nutrient content that possess functional properties (i.e., microorganisms such as Lactobacillus).

Genistein is one of the most well-researched isoflavones (a group of flavonoid compounds belonging to the larger class of phytochemicals called phenols—see definition on page 240). Noted as one of the primary isoflavones in soybeans, soy foods are the richest dietary source of genistein. Health benefits linked to genistein and other isoflavones include protection against certain types of cancers, heart disease and osteoporosis.

Glutathione is an antioxidant made up of the linked amino acids glutamic acid, cysteine and glycine. It is synthesized in plant and animal. As part of the selenium-containing enzyme glutathione peroxidase, it works in concert with Vitamin E to prevent the production of free radical chain reactions. This water-soluble substance is found in onions and potatoes, as well as other fruits and vegetables. It has also exhibited the promising effect of detoxifying cancer-causing substances.

Glycosylation is a process with a variety of different mechanisms, where glucose molecules attach to different proteins in the bloodstream. This process makes the protein stiff and inflexible. In diabetes, sugar molecules attach to hemoglobin blood proteins. An accumulation of glycated hemoglobin proteins is thought to damage blood vessels in the body, especially in the kidneys and the eyes, causing the common diabetic complications of kidney failure and blindness.

HDL cholesterol—often referred to as "good" cholesterol or "Highly Desirable" cholesterol—is a high-density lipoprotein that transports cholesterol from cells to the liver, where the cholesterol is either recycled or disposed of. High blood levels of HDL cholesterol are associated with lower risk of heart attack, a protective effect.

Indoles are organosulfur compounds formed from glucosinolates substances found in cruciferous vegetables, namely Brussels sprouts, rutabaga and mustard greens. They have been linked with cancer prevention due to their ability to help favorably alter carcinogen metabolism, and they may also lower blood cholesterol.

Indole-3-carbinol is a member of the indole group, a class of organosulfur compound phytochemicals. Studies have indicated indole-3-carbinol may help protect against estrogen-related cancers, such as breast cancer, and may also help lower cholesterol.

Inositol hexaphosphate is another name for the phytochemical phytate (see definition on page 240).

Isoflavones. These plant substances are a subclass of flavonoids, which belong to an even larger group of phytochemicals, called phenols (see definition on page 240). The most widely recognized isoflavones include genistein and diadzein. The richest dietary source of isoflavones is soy foods (i.e., soybeans, soy flour, tofu, soymilk, etc.). Soy products vary in their content of isoflavones, and processing also affects this. Scientific attention to isoflavones has peaked recently, with studies indicating that these plant substances may have a potential role in prevention and treatment of various chronic diseases as they have shown to impact metabolic and biological body functions. Also referred to as phytoestrogens (meaning "plant estrogens"), isoflavones have demonstrated the ability to block human estrogens by tying up estrogen receptors on cells and thus affect hormone-related cancers, including breast and prostate cancer. Current research has also demonstrated promising effects of isoflavones with respect to heart disease due to their roles as antioxidants. They possess the ability to decrease unfavorable oxidation of LDL cholesterol and help prevent damage to blood vessels. Isoflavones are also under investigation regarding their potential to protect against osteoporosis and minimize menopause symptoms.

Isothiocyanates are organosulfur compounds formed from glucosinolate substances found in cruciferous vegetables. This group of phytochemicals has demonstrated potent anticancer activity in research.

Kaempherol is a flavonoid (belonging to the larger class of phytochemicals called phenols) found mostly in fruits and vegetables that has demonstrated antioxidant activity (see flavonoid definition on page 236).

LDL cholesterol—commonly referred to as "bad" cholesterol or "Least Desirable" cholesterol—is a low-density lipoprotein that circulates throughout the body delivering its contents of cholesterol and triglycerides to cells. Elevated LDL concentrations in the blood are associated with increased damage to blood vessels and promotion of heart disease.

Lignans are plant substances that belong to the group of phytochemicals called phenols. They are also considered phytoestrogens as they can be converted to plant estrogen by fermentation in the intestines. Research has shown that lignans have key antioxidant properties. Lignans may favorably affect hormone-related cancers as the weak estrogens they contain may occupy the estrogen receptors on cells, thus inhibiting the growth of estrogen stimulated tumors, such as breast cancer. Flaxseed is the richest source of lignans, and other foods that supply them in smaller amounts include whole grains, soybeans and some berries and vegetables.

Limonene is a monoterpene substance (belonging to the larger phytochemical class called terpenes (see definition on page 242) that is found in the oils of citrus peels and many herbs such as caraway, coriander, dill and fennel. Research has indicated that limonene may have cancer-preventative activity.

Lutein is a member of the carotenoid class of phytochemicals that has demonstrated powerful antioxidant activity and is key to maintenance of vision. Lutein is one of the two carotenoids found in the eye and is believed to protect against cataracts and development of age-related macular degeneration. Rich food sources of lutein are green vegetables such as kale, spinach and avocado.

Lycopene is a member of the carotenoid class of phytochemicals that has potent antioxidant effects. Found primarily in tomato and tomato products, as well as grapefruit and watermelon, this substance has been currently researched in the area of prostate cancer prevention.

Monoterpenes are a group of compounds belonging to the larger class of phytochemicals called terpenes (see definition on page 242). Examples of monoterpenes include limonene and perillyl alcohol found in the oils of citrus peels and a variety of herbs. These compounds have exhibited promising anticancer and cardio-protective effects in recent research.

Monounsaturated fat is a type of fatty acid that is liquid at room temperature and is named for or classified by its particular chemical structure. Generally all fatty acids are chains of carbon and hydrogen atoms with an acid (containing oxygen) attached. A monounsaturated acid has two of the hydrogens in the chain missing, which leads to a change in its arrangement, creating one double bond. Key food sources of monounsaturated fats are plant foods such as olive, peanut and canola oil, as well as avocado. Monounsaturated fats have the beneficial effect of lowering blood cholesterol.

Nitrates and nitrites are substances added to food to preserve color, enhance flavor and decrease bacterial growth. Though these additives have beneficial effects on food quality, they can be converted in the body to cancer-causing substances called nitrosamines when mixed with the acid of the stomach. Nitrites are found in smoked, cured and fermented foods. Nitrates are found naturally in some foods and can be changed to nitrites by bacteria in the mouth. Vitamins C and E and phytochemicals can block the formation of nitrosamines.

Omega-3 fatty acids are polyunsaturated fatty acids in which the "3" denotes the position of the first double bond (3 carbon atoms from one of its ends). Linolenic acid is the primary member of the omega-3 family, which can be used by the body to make two other key omega fatty acids, named eicosapentaenoic acid and docosahexaenoic acid, needed for body tissues such as the brain and eyes. Linolenic acid is considered "essential" because the body cannot make it, and therefore it must be supplied by diet. (As stated above, once given linoleic acid, the body can make the other fatty acids, yet the conversion process is often slow so it is more effective to obtain them from foods.) Key food sources of omega-3 fatty acids include fish, such as tuna, salmon and mackerel, as well as nuts, seeds, soybeans and vegetable oils. Omega-3 fatty acids are needed for normal growth and development and may play an important role in the prevention and treatment of coronary artery disease, hypertension, diabetes, arthritis, other inflammatory and autoimmune disorders, and cancer.

Omega-6 fatty acids are polyunsaturated fatty acids in which the "6" denotes the position of the first double bond (6 carbon atoms from one of its ends). Linoleic acid is the primary member of the omega-6 family, which the body can use to synthesize another important fatty acid called arachidonic acid that is key to maintaining the structure and function of cell membranes. Like the omega-3 linolenic fatty acid, linoleic acid is also considered "essential" because the body cannot make it, and therefore it must be supplied by diet. (As stated above, once given linolenic acid, the body can make arachidonic acid, yet the conversion process is often slow so it is more effective to obtain it from foods.) The main dietary sources to obtain omega-6 fatty acids are vegetable oils, such as corn, safflower, soybean, sesame and sunflower oils.

Organosulfides, a major class of phytochemicals including indoles, dithiolithones, thiocynates and isothiocyanates, are present in cruciferous vegetables and other allium compounds found in onions and garlic. These various substances have demonstrated many beneficial effects in recent research. Dithiolithiones, such as sulforophane and indoles, work primarily against cancer. Allium compounds, namely diallyl sulfide, have also been linked to cancer prevention and promotion of heart health.

Oxidation is the chemical combination of a substance with oxygen. In the body, highly reactive free radical forms of oxygen can attach to other compounds in cells, causing structural damage to cell protein, fats or DNA material. Polyunsaturated fat molecules in cell membranes and LDL cholesterol are particularly susceptible to free radical damage by oxidation. For example, the oxidized form of LDL cholesterol changes readily into substances that contribute to lesions in blood vessel walls, building up as plaque that gradually shrinks the circumference of the vessels and makes them less flexible. Antioxidants can help neutralize free radicals and prevent oxidation.

Oxidative balance is the dynamic balance between the antioxidant system and the production of reactive oxygen species (or free radicals) in the body. Oxidative stress occurs when this equilibrium shifts in favor of free radicals or pro-oxidants.

Perillyl alcohol is a monoterpene substance (belonging to the larger phytochemical class called terpenes—see definition on page 242) that is found in the oils of citrus peels, cherries and many herbs such as spearmint and sage. Research has indicated that perillyl alcohol may have cancer-preventative activity.

Phenolic compounds are the largest group of phytochemicals (as many as 8000 identified) that are present in variable amounts in virtually all plant foods, such as cereals, vegetables, fruits, legumes, nuts, teas and cocoa. Recent interest in phenols has surged due to their potential health benefits that include antioxidant activity and anti-cancer and anti-inflammatory effects. Well-studied groups of phenols include flavonoids and phenolic acids.

Phytic acid/phytate is a phytochemical found in whole grains, beans (soybeans), nuts and seeds. Though phytate may decrease the availability of minerals in these foods, research has demonstrated it has many beneficial health effects such as inhibiting the formation of cancer and assisting in controlling blood sugar, cholesterol and triglycerides.

Phytochemicals are organic components of plants that have come to be recognized as physiologically-active substances with health-promoting and protecting properties. ("Phyto" originates from a Greek word meaning "plant.") Thousands of different phytochemicals have been identified in a wide variety of plant foods, such as fruits, vegetables, legumes, whole grains, nuts and seeds. Examples of major classes of phytochemicals include carotenoids and phenols. Unlike the nutrients protein, fat, vitamins and minerals, phytochemicals are currently not deemed as "essential" for life, though some references are made with the term "phytonutrient." Many promising and beneficial effects have been linked to phytochemicals, namely in the areas of cardiovascular disease, cancer and anti-aging research. The mechanisms of action by which these plant substances produce their effects are still subject to much scientific investigation.

Phytoestrogens are estrogens found in plants that are weaker than human estrogen but still have shown to impact metabolic and biological body functions. Studies have indicated they possess the ability to block estrogens by tying up estrogen receptors on cells, thereby affecting hormone-related cancers, including breast and prostate cancer. Recent research has also demonstrated promising effects of phytoestrogens with respect to heart disease and osteoporosis protection. Key phytoestrogen examples are isoflavones and lignans, which are found in soy products as well as in flaxseed.

Phytostanol—also known as plant stanols—are thought to contribute to lowering total and LDL cholesterol levels. Plant stanols are natural substances found in nuts, vegetable oils, corn, rice, and some other plants. Plant stanols are similar in structure to cholesterol, which enables them to effectively compete for and inhibit cholesterol absorption, thereby causing it to be discarded from the body. They appear to be equal in efficacy to phytosterols.

Phytosterols are plant sterols that are natural dietary components. The most common plant sterols are ß-sitosterol, campesterol and stigmasterol. Key food sources include nuts (almonds, cashews, peanuts), seeds (sesame, sunflower), whole wheat, corn, soybeans and many vegetable oils. Aside from these natural sources, plant sterols such as sitosterol have been added to margarine for their beneficial health effects. Recent studies show that these plant substances are effective in lowering cholesterol because they have structure similar to human cholesterol. This structural property enables phytosterols to effectively compete for and inhibit cholesterol absorption, thereby causing it to be discarded from the body. Research has also indicated that phytosterols have antioxidant activity and may provide protection against cancer, namely colon cancer.

Polyunsaturated fats are a type of fatty acids that are liquid at room temperature and are named for or classified by their particular chemical structure. Generally all fatty acids are chains of carbon and hydrogen atoms with an acid (containing oxygen) attached. A polyunsaturated acid lacks four or more hydrogens in the chain, which leads to a change in its arrangement such that at least two double bonds are formed. The omega-fatty acids (see definition on page 239) are part of this class. Dietary sources of polyunsaturated fatty acids are found in plant foods such as walnuts and oils (safflower, sunflower, soybean), as well as in seafood. Beneficial health effects from consumption of polyunsaturated fats may include the lowering of blood cholesterol and cancer prevention, which is specifically linked to the omega-fatty acids.

Pro-oxidant is any substance that promotes or increases oxidation. Examples of oxidants include chemicals, sunlight and dietary sources (such as certain types of fats). If excessive, the production of oxidants and free radicals can be harmful to the body, causing cellular damage leading to degenerative disease.

Protease inhibitors are phytochemicals that are widely distributed in plants, namely seeds, legumes (i.e., soybeans) and green vegetables. Trypsin inhibitors, found in spinach and broccoli, are a subset of this class of compounds and have been well researched. Protection against cancer is a beneficial effect of protease inhibitors that has been demonstrated in preliminary studies.

Quercetin is one of the most widely researched flavonoid compounds (belonging to the larger class of phytochemicals—called phenols). This substance is found in highest concentration in onions, apples, grapes and broccoli. It has demonstrated key antioxidant activity in research and more specifically has the potential to decrease inflammation, inhibit cancer formation and protect against the development of atherosclerosis.

Resveratrol is a substance belonging to the flavonoid group of phytochemicals, which are part of an even larger class of phytochemicals—called phenols. Found primarily in the skins of grapes (along with grape juice and wine), resveratrol has been linked to key health benefits including reduction of heart disease and cancer risk.

Retinol is another name for fat-soluble Vitamin A. It functions in vision as an essential constituent of the visual pigments of the eyes and also plays an important role in growth, bone development and the maintenance of healthy mucous membranes. Preformed Vitamin A occurs only in foods of animal origin and pill supplements. Plants, namely the carotenoids (i.e., beta-carotene) contain provitamin A, a form that can be converted to Vitamin A in the body once consumed. Pro-vitamin A is found primarily in fruits and vegetables of green and orange color, such as spinach, broccoli, carrots and sweet potato.

Saponins are plant substances found in beans, nuts, whole grains and selected herbs. This group of phytochemicals has been reported to potentially protect against cancer and heart disease.

Selenium is a trace element that functions as part of an antioxidant enzyme compound, glutathione peroxidase. This compound works in concert with Vitamin E to block the production of free radical chain reactions. It helps to protect polyunsaturated fatty acids from unfavorable oxidation. Foods rich in selenium include garlic, Brazil nuts and grains.

Silymarin is a flavonoid (belonging to the larger class of phytochemicals called phenols) that has shown promising effects in recent research in treating liver disease. Aside from protecting against liver toxicity in animal studies, this substance has demonstrated potent antioxidant activity and may play a cancer-protective role. Silymarin is found in vegetables such as artichokes.

Sitosterol is a plant substance belonging to the group of phytochemicals called phytosterols, which is similar in structure to cholesterol. It is believed that moderate levels of consumption of sitosterol can interfere with cholesterol absorption and result in decreased serum cholesterol levels. Plant sources are beans and oils.

Stigmasterol is a plant substance belonging to the group of phytochemicals called phytosterols, which is similar in structure to cholesterol. It is believed that moderate levels of consumption of stigmasterol can interfere with cholesterol absorption and result in decreased serum cholesterol levels. Plant sources are beans and oils.

Terpenes/terpenoids are a broad class of phytochemicals found in a wide variety of herbs. Monoterpenes (i.e., limonene and perillyl alcohol) and triterpenes are subgroups that have been well studied. Research has indicated that these plant substances are key antioxidants and have protective effects against cancer and heart disease.

Vanillin is a phenolic compound found in vanilla beans and cloves that has shown to inhibit cancer and atherosclerosis in recent research (see definition for phenols on page 240).

Vitamin C is a water-soluble vitamin and antioxidant that functions in the synthesis of the structural protein collagen, which gives strength and elasticity to the skin, and maintains the integrity of blood vessels, bones and teeth. This vitamin is also important for wound healing, immune function, amino acid metabolism and iron absorption. Major food sources include citrus and tropical fruits, cruciferous and dark green vegetables, strawberries and melons.

Vitamin E is a fat-soluble vitamin and key antioxidant which protects cell membranes and blood cells. It also prevents unfavorable oxidation of polyunsaturated fatty acids and other fats. Foods rich in Vitamin E are vegetable oils, whole grains, nuts and seeds.

Zeaxanthin is a member of the carotenoid class of phytochemicals that has demonstrated powerful antioxidant activity and is key to maintenance of vision. Zeaxanthin is one of the two carotenoids found in the eye (lutein is the second) and is believed to protect against development of cataracts and age-related macular degeneration. Rich food sources of zeaxanthin are green vegetables and citrus fruits.

Index

African Groundnut Stew, 179–80

Aging and food, 7

Alpha-linolenic acid (ALA), 90, 189, 204

Alpha-tocopherol, 126

Amber Ginger Ale, 85–86

Angiogenesis, 108

Anthocyanin, 22

Antiaging:
    defined, 6
    foods, 11–19
    medicine, 2

Antioxidants, 11–12, 72, 124, 206
    foods high in, list, 12–14

Asian Chicken Salad, 96–98

Astaxanthin, 191

Avocado, 87–88
    recipes for, 90–91

Baba Ghanouj, 73–75

Baby Boomers, 1–2

Banana-Caramel "Ice Cream" with Toasted Walnuts, 215–16

Banana-Fudge Smoothie, 122

Beans, 165–68

Beets, 124–25
    recipes for, 130–31

Bell pepper, 125
    recipes for, 127–28, 132–33, 138

Bengali Breakfast Grains, 156–57

Bengali Carrot Sauté, 133–35

Benign prostatic hyperplasia, 147

Berries, 22–23
    recipes for, 28–39

Beta-carotene, 55–56

Betaine, 124–25

Black bean, 167
    Dumplings, Tiny Chinese, 169–71
    recipes for, 169–71, 175–76

Blackberry Mint Sorbet, 38–39

Black tea, 206–7
    Chicken with Ginger and Mint, 209–10

Blood glucose, 10–11

Blueberry, 22
    Banana Muffins, 31–33
    Upside-Down Clafouti, 34–35

Boron, 21

Bowerman, Susan, 88

Brazil nuts, 204

Breakfast Grains:
    Bengali, 156–57
    Warm, with Dried Cherries and Toasted Pecans, 30–31

Broccoli-Dill Soup with Lemon and Tahini, 91–92

Brussels Sprouts, Nutty Glazed, 104–5

Buckwheat, 146

Bulgur, 144
    Casbah, 150–51

recipes for, 150–51, 156–57, 163–64

Butyrate, 168

Cancer, 42, 56, 72–73, 88, 108, 123, 145–46, 167–68, 189–90, 206

Cannellini beans, 167–68
    recipes for, 172–76

Caponata, 210–12

Cara's Ginger Crackers, 161–62

Caribbean Salmon Croquettes, 192–93

Caribbean Sweet Potatoes, 135–36

Carotenoids, 42, 124–25

Carrot, 123–24
    recipes for, 133–35
    Sauté, Bengali, 133–34

Casbah Bulgur, 150–51

Casey's Pumpkin Soup, 128–29

Chicken, 189
    Black Tea with Ginger and Mint, 209–10
    Grilled Miso, 115–16
    Grilled with Walnut and Pomegranate Sauce, 207–9
    Mole with Pumpkin and Sesame Seeds, 148-49
    Savory Tagine with Slivered Dried Plums and Baby Artichokes, 26-27

Chicken (*cont.*)
  Shwarma in Warm Pitas with
    Tomato-Cucumber Salad,
    78–79
Chickpea, 166–67
  Crêpes, 182–83
  recipes for, 171–72, 174–75,
    177–78, 182–83
Chocolate, 205, 212
  Caramel Pudding, 121–22
  Mexican Hot, 216–17
Cholesterol, 87–88, 204
Citrus, 41–42
  recipes for, 44–48
Clafouti, Blueberry Upside-Down,
    34–35
Cocoa, 19, 204–5
  powder, 19
  recipes for, 210–12, 216–17
Cold water fish, 187–89
Compote, Warm Blueberry,
    37–38
Confit, Red Pepper, 138
Cookies
  PB&J Granola Bars, 50–51
  Spicy Ginger-Berry Biscotti,
    84–85
Corn, 144
  recipes for, 151–52, 160–61
Coumarin, 42
Crackers, Cara's Ginger, 161–62
Cranberries, 23
Cranberry Spice Jam, 33–34
Creamy Chickpea and Lentil Stew
    with Caramelized Onions,
    171–72
Creamy Hummus, 110–11
Creamy Onion Soup with Roasted
    Garlic and Thyme, 75–76
Creamy Spinach with Peppery
    Cheese, 98–99
Creamy Stone-Ground Polenta,
    151–52
Crêpes, Chickpea, 182–83

Crispy Cornmeal Waffles with
    Warm Berry Syrup, 28–29
Crispy Kale Croquettes, 101–2
Crispy Vegetarian Spring Rolls
    with Shanghai Plum Sauce,
    24–26
Croquettes
  Caribbean Salmon, 192–93
  Crispy Kale, 101–2
Cruciferous vegetables, 89
  recipes for, 96–98, 100, 104–5
Curry
  Chicken Stew, 76–77
  Creamed Cabbage, 100
  Roasted Tomato with Gingered
    Garbanzo Beans and Baby
    Spinach, 63–65

Daidzein, 108
Davies, Kelvin, Dr., 8
DHEA (dehydroepiandrosterone),
    10
Dried plums, 21–22
Drinks
  Amber Ginger Ale, 85–86
  Banana Fudge Smoothie, 122
  Masala Chai, 217–18
  Mexican Hot Chocolate, 216–17
  Moroccan Mint Tea, 219
  Mulled Red Wine, 52–53
  Stop the Clock! Cranberry-
    Grape, 48–49
  Sweet Mango Lassi, 140–41
Dumplings, Tiny Chinese Black
    Bean, 169–71
Dutching process, 205

Edamame, 109
  Guacamole, 111–12
Eggplant
  Egyptian Salad, 94–96
  Roasted Purée, 73–75
  Roasted Salad, 210–12
Ellagic acid, 23

Endothelin-1, 43
Enzymes, 9–10
Epicatechin, 205
Epigallocatechin gallate, 206, 214
Essential fatty acids (EFAs), 187
Estrogen, 108, 189–90
Etouffée, Three-Fish with Baby
    Artichokes and Spicy
    Tomato Broth, 190–91

Falafel Sandwiches, 177–78
Fava bean, 166
  recipes for, 181–82
  Stew, 181–82
Fiber, 42, 125
Fish, 187–89
  recipes for, 190–98
Flavonoids, 42–43, 205–6
Flax, 189–90
  recipes for, 199–201
Flaxjacks, Whole-Grain,
    199–200
Foods
  antiaging, 11–19
  citrus and grapes, 41–54
  cocoa powder, 19
  ginger, onion, and garlic, 71–86
  grains and seeds, 143–64
  greens, 87–105
  high in antioxidants, list, 12–14
  nutrient-poor, 10
  olive oil, 18
  pantry of, 15–16
  plums and berries, 21–39
  recommendations for, 16
  red and yellow fruits and
    vegetables, 123–41
  sorghum syrup, 17
  soy, 107–22
  tomatoes, 55–69
Foul, 181–82
Free radicals, 8–9, 124
French paradox, 43
French Toast, Lemony, 200–201

Garbanzo beans. *See* Chickpeas
Garlic, 73
    recipes for, 73–83
    Roasted Purée, 82–83
Genistein, 108
Ginger, 71–72
    Ale, Amber, 85–86
    Berry Biscotti, Spicy, 84–85
    Crackers, Cara's, 161–62
    Preserved, 83–84
    recipes for, 76–78, 83–86
Gingerol, 72
Glucose, 10–11
Glutathione transferase, 42
Gluten, 144
Glycosylation, 10
G6PD-deficiency, 166
Grainola, Stop the Clock!, 157–58
Grains, 143–46
    recipes for, 150–64
Grapes, 42–44
    recipes for, 48–53
Greens, 87–90
    recipes for, 90–105
Green tea, 206–7
    Sorbet with Candied Ginger
        and Toasted Walnuts,
        213–14
Grilled Chicken with Walnut and
        Pomegranate Sauce, 207–9
Grilled Miso Chicken, 115–16
Guacamole, 87–88

Harira with Roasted Vegetables,
        117–18
Harman, Denham, Dr., 8
Health promotion, rules for, 2
Heart disease, 22, 43, 204–5
Heber, David, Dr., 56
Hippocrates, 169
Homocysteine, 125
Honey, dark, 17
Hormones, 188–89
Hummus, Creamy, 110–11

Icy Gazpacho with Fresh Lime and
        Corn Tortilla Spikes, 59–60
Immune system, 73
Indoles, 89
Inflammation, 10
Isoflavones, 108–9
Isothiocyanates, 89
Italian Bean and Sauerkraut Soup,
        172–73

Jam
    Cranberry Spice, 33–34
    Tomato with Lemon and Basil,
        67–68
Jelly, Purple Grape, 49–50
Jota, 172–73
Juice, Stop the Clock! Cranberry-
        Grape, 48–49

Kaempherol, 42
Kasha, 146

LDL (low-density lipoprotein), 22
L-dopa, 182
Legumes, 165–69
    recipes for, 169–85
Lemon Tahini Sauce, 46–47
Lemony French Toast, 200–201
Lentils, 169
    recipes for, 171–72, 184–85
    Stovetop Barbecue, 184–85
Lettuce, 90
    recipes for, 94–96
Lignans, 144, 189–90
Limonene, 42
Low-calorie diet, 10
Luteolin, 42
Lycopene, 55–57
Lysine, 147

Maccha, 213–14
Macular degeneration, 42, 56–57, 88
Mahogany Millet with Kasha,
        Dried Blueberries, Mango,

    and Toasted Walnuts,
        152–53
Mango, 126
    recipes for, 140–41
Masala Chai, 217–18
Menopause, 108
Messina, Mark, Dr., 109
Metabolism, 9
Mexican Hot Chocolate, 216–17
Millet, 146
    Mahogany, with Kasha, Dried
        Blueberries, Mango, and
        Toasted Walnuts, 152–53
    recipes for, 152–53
Miso, 109–10
    Rice Porridge, 119
    Soup with Wilted Greens
        and Roasted Tomatoes,
        114–15
Moroccan Beet Salad, 130–31
Moroccan Mint Tea, 219
Moussaka, Savory with Pumate
        Béchamel, 65–67
Muffins, Blueberry Banana,
        31–33
Mulled Red Wine, 52–53
Mustard Greens, Southern-Style,
        103–4

Neurotransmitters, 204
Nutrient density, 10
Nutrient-poor foods, 10
Nuts, 203–4
    recipes for, 207–9, 212–13, 215–16
Nutty Glazed Brussels Sprouts,
        104–5
Nutty Tomato Pesto, 212–13

Oats, 144
    recipes for, 157–58
Old-Fashioned Orange Sherbet,
        120–21
Olive oil, 18
Omega-3 fatty acids, 188–89

Onions, 72–73
    Caramelized, with Scalloped
        Tomatoes, 80–81
    recipes for, 75–81
ORAC measurement, 11–14
Oxidation, 9
Oxidative stress, 9–11
Oxygen paradox, 8

Panch Puran, 133, 135
Pan-Roasted Salmon with Wilted
    Chard and Tomato-Mint
    Raita, 194–96
Pantry, 15–16
PB&J Granola Bars, 50–51
Peanut, 168
    African Groundnut Stew,
        179–80
    recipes for, 179–80
Pectin, 42, 125
PEITC (phenyl ethyl
    isothiocyanate), 89
Perricone, Nicholas, Dr., 10–11
The Perricone Prescription
    (Perricone), 10
Persian Vegetable Stew, 174–75
Pesto, Nutty Tomato, 212–13
Phenolic compounds, 22
Phytic acid, 108
Phytochemicals, 11, 108
Phytoestrogens, 108
Phytosterols, 88, 108, 168
Pita Bread, Whole-Wheat,
    154–55
Platelet aggregation, 204
Plums, 21–22
    recipes for, 24–27
Polenta, Creamy Stone-Ground,
    151–52
Polyphenols, 43
Pomegranate, 209
Poppy seed, 163–64
    Porridge, Lemony, 163–64

Porridge
    Kutia (Lemony Poppy Seed),
        163–64
    Miso Rice, 119
Prebiotics, 167
Preserved Ginger, 83–84
Preserved Lemons, 47–48
Prior, Ronald, Dr., 11
Proanthocyanidins, 23
Probiotics, 110
Procyandin, 205
Prolla, Tomas, Dr., 10
Protease inhibitors, 144, 167
Pudding
    Chocolate-Caramel, 121–22
    Indian, 160–61
Pumpkin, 125
    Butter, 139–40
    recipes for, 128–29, 139–40
    seeds, 147
Purple Grape Jelly, 49–50
Purple grapes, 42–43

Quercetin, 72, 88

Raspberries, 23
Recipes:
    berry, 28–39
    citrus, 44–48
    cocoa, 210–12, 216–17
    fish, 190–98
    flax, 199–201
    garlic, 73–83
    ginger, 76–78, 83–86
    grains and seeds, 148–64
    grape, 48–53
    greens, 90–105
    nut, 207–9, 212–13, 215–16
    onion, 75–81
    plum, 24–27
    red and yellow vegetables and
        fruit, 127–41
    soy, 110–22

    tea, 209–10, 213–14, 217–19
    tomato, 57–69
Red Pepper Confit, 138
Red wine grape, 43–44
Resistant starch, 167–68
Resveratrol, 44
Rhamnetin, 94
Richardson, Alexandra, 189
Roasted Eggplant Purée, 73–75
Roasted Eggplant Salad, 210–12
Roasted Garlic Purée, 82–83
Roasted Pepper Soup, 127–28
Roasted Sweet Potatoes with
    Rosemary, 137
Roasted Tomato Curry with
    Gingered Garbanzo Beans
    and Baby Spinach, 63–65
Rutin, 146

Saag Paneer, 98–99
Salad
    Asian Chicken, 96–98
    Egyptian Eggplant, 94–96
    Moroccan Beet, 130–31
    Roasted Eggplant, 210–12
    Romesco, 132–33
    Succotash, 175–76
    Sweet and Spicy Orange, 44–45
    Watercress and Cranberry, with
        Roasted Onion Dressing,
        93–94
Salade Romesco, 132–33
Salmon
    Caribbean Croquettes, 192–93
    Charmoula, 196–97
    Pan-Roasted with Wilted Chard
        and Tomato-Mint Raita,
        194–96
Sandwich
    Chicken Shwarma in Warm
        Pitas with Tomato-
        Cucumber Salad, 78–79
    Falafel, 177–78

Saponins, 108–9, 169
Sassy Tomato-Avocado Soup, 90–91
Sauce
    Charmoula, 196–97
    Lemon Tahini, 46–47
    Southwestern Barbecue with
        Chipotle Chiles, 68–69
    Tangy Mustard-Tahini, 159
    Walnut and Pomegranate, 207–9
Savory Chicken Tagine with
    Slivered Dried Plums and
    Baby Artichokes, 26–27
Savory Moussaka with Pumate
    Béchamel, 65–67
Scalloped Tomatoes with
    Caramelized Onions, 80–81
Seeds, 147
    recipes for, 148–49, 157–59,
        161–64
Selenium, 204
Serotonin, 204
Sesame seeds, 147
    recipes for, 159
Sherbet, Old-Fashioned Orange,
    120–21
Shogaol, 72
Sinigrin, 105
Skin wrinkles, 10–11, 56
Smoky Tomato Stew with Country
    Bread and Cannellini
    Beans, 62–63
Smoothie, Banana-Fudge, 122
Socca, 182–83
Sorbet
    Blackberry Mint, 38–39
    Green Tea with Candied Ginger
        and Toasted Walnuts,
        213–14
Sorbitol, 22
Sorghum
    grain, 146
    recipes for, 154–55, 161–62
    syrup, 17

Soup
    Broccoli-Dill, with Lemon and
        Tahini, 91–92
    Casey's Pumpkin, 128–29
    Creamy Onion with Roasted
        Garlic and Thyme, 75–76
    Icy Gazpacho with Fresh Lime
        and Corn Tortilla Spikes,
        59–60
    Italian Bean and Sauerkraut,
        172–73
    Miso, with Wilted Greens and
        Roasted Tomatoes, 114–15
    Roasted Pepper, 127–28
    Sassy Tomato-Avocado, 90–91
    Tomato-Ginger Bisque, 60–61
    Tomato-Lentil, 57–58
Southern Style Mustard Greens,
    103–4
Southwestern Barbecue Sauce with
    Chipotle Chiles, 68–69
Soy, 107–10
    recipes for, 110–22
Soymilk, 109
Spicy Fish Stew, 197–98
Spicy Ginger-Berry Biscotti, 84–85
Spinach, 88–89
    Creamy with Peppery Cheese,
        98–99
    recipes for, 98–99
Spring Rolls, Crispy Vegetarian
    with Shanghai Plum Sauce,
    24–26
Stew
    African Groundnut, 179–80
    Creamy Chickpea and Lentil
        with Caramelized Onions,
        171–72
    Curried Chicken, 76–77
    Fava Bean, 181–82
    Harira with Roasted Vegetables,
        117–18
    Persian Vegetable, 174–75

Smoky Tomato with Country
    Bread and Cannellini
    Beans, 62–63
Spicy Fish, 197–98
Three-Fish Etouffée with Baby
    Artichokes and Spicy
    Tomato Broth, 190–91
Stop the Clock! Cranberry-Grape
    Juice, 48–49
Stop the Clock! Grainola, 157–58
Stop the Clock! Trail Mix, 113
Stovetop Barbecued Lentils, 184–85
Strawberry, 23
    Gelée, 36–37
Succotash Salad, 175–76
Sugars, 10–11, 17
Sulfonate, 72
Sweet and Spicy Orange Salad,
    44–45
Sweet Mango Lassi, 140–41
Sweet potatoes, 126
    Caribbean, 135–36
    recipes for, 135–37
    Roasted, with Rosemary, 137

Tangy Mustard-Tahini Sauce,
    159
Tea, 206–7
    recipes for, 209–10, 213–14,
        217–19
Three-Fish Etouffée with Baby
    Artichokes and Spicy
    Tomato Broth, 190–91
Tiny Chinese Black Bean
    Dumplings, 169–71
Tofu, 110
Tomato, 55–57
    Ginger Bisque, 60–61
    Jam with Lemon and Basil,
        67–68
    Lentil Soup, 57–58
    recipes for, 57–69
Trail Mix, Stop the Clock!, 113

Ultraviolet rays, 56–57
USDA (United States Department of Agriculture), 11

Violaxanthin, 126
Vitamin A, 124
Vitamin C, 125

Waffles, Crispy Cornmeal with Warm Berry Syrup, 28–29

Warm Blueberry Compote, 37–38
Warm Breakfast Grains with Dried Cherries and Toasted Pecans, 30–31
Watercress, 89–90
and Cranberry Salad with Roasted Onion Dressing, 93–94
recipes for, 93–94
Weindruch, Richard, Dr., 10

Wheat, 145
recipes for, 154–55, 161–62
Whole-Grain Flaxjacks, 199–200
Whole-Wheat Pita Bread, 154–55
Wine, Mulled Red, 52–53
The Wrinkle Cure (Perricone), 10

Xeaxanthin, 144

Zingerone, 72